THE CITY & GUILDS A-Z
BEAUTY THERAPY

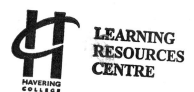

LEARNING
RESOURCES
CENTRE

HAVERING
COLLEGE

About City & Guilds

City & Guilds is the UK's leading provider of vocational qualifications, offering over 500 awards across a wide range of industries and progressing from entry level to the highest levels of professional achievement. With over 8500 centres in 100 countries, City & Guilds is recognised by employers worldwide for providing qualifications that offer proof of the skills they need to get the job done.

Equal opportunities

City & Guilds fully supports the principle of equal opportunities and we are committed to satisfying this principle in all our activities and published material. A copy of our equal opportunities policy statement is available on the City & Guilds website.

First edition 2012

ISBN 978 0 85193 224 8

Edited by Rachel Howells
Designed and typeset by Select Typesetters Ltd
Printed in the UK by Swallowtail Print

Publications

For information about or to order City & Guilds support materials, contact 0844 534 0000 or centresupport@cityandguilds.com. You can find more information about the materials we have available at www.cityandguilds.com/publications.

Every effort has been made to ensure that the information contained in this publication is true and correct at the time of going to press. However, City & Guilds' products and services are subject to continuous development and improvement, and the right is reserved to change products and services from time to time. City & Guilds cannot accept liability for loss or damage arising from the use of information in this publication.

City & Guilds
1 Giltspur Street
London EC1A 9DD

T 0844 543 0033
www.cityandguilds.com
publishingfeedback@cityandguilds.com

CONTENTS

Acknowledgements   **04**

Introduction – how to use this book   **05**

The City & Guilds A–Z   **06**

ACKNOWLEDGEMENTS

Every effort has been made to acknowledge all copyright holders as below and the publishers will, if notified, correct any errors in future editions.

City & Guilds would like to sincerely thank the following:
For invaluable beauty therapy expertise Sarah Farrell and Anita Crosland.

For providing pictures:
Alexandra House Spa, Huddersfield: p108; **Andover College:** pp41, 82, 84, 99, 113; **Annemarie Borlind – Beautiful Naturally:** p83; **Baglioni Spa by SPC (www.baglionispa.co.uk):** p113; **Barry Craig:** p67; **Bluestone National Park Resort:** pp121, 137; **Bobbi Brown:** p108; **Bournemouth and Poole College:** pp51, 56; **Buttercups Uniforms:** p74; **Carlton Group:** pp15, 20, 45, 49, 53, 61, 111; **Carlton Professional:** p136; **Central Sussex College:** pp27, 32, 35, 37, 41, 55, 67, 70, 79, 86, 89, 106, 129, 134; **Central Training Group:** p6, 121; **Champneys Health Resorts (www.champneys.com):** pp34, 42, 105, 109, 120, 122; **Collin UK:** p21; **Derby College:** p46, 82; **Dermacolor:** p34; **Dermalogica:** pp51, 87; **Desmond Murray:** p133; **Elemis:** p27; **Ellisons:** pp16, 99, 116; **Ergoline UK:** p125; **EzFlow:** p111; **Folkestone Academy:** p57; **Fotolia:** p43; **Getty Images/Comstock Images:** p13; **Goddess International:** p20; **Habia:** pp62, 62; **Havering College:** pp43, 112; **Hebe:** pp16, 28, 45, 51, 54, 67, 122, 136; **Hertford Regional College:** pp13, 28, 33, 37, 41, 45, 51, 67, 78, 81, 91, 96, 102, 103, 125; **IIAA College Programme:** p127; **iStockphoto.com:** © ampyang p30, © andipantz p29, © Andrew J Shearer p24, © angelhell p12, © Cathy Britcliffe p39, © Chris Gramly p53, © claire222 p124, © comotion_design p110, © comotion_design p120, © Dana Bartekoske p132, © diego_cervo p10, © DIGIcal p134, © DomenicoGelermo p72, © drbimages p71, © Dr Bouz p76, © edufentesg p64, © Farina2000 p9, © fatbob2 p110, © FotoShoot p52, © George Peters p22, © hartphotography1 p47, © iconogenic pp12, 28, 31, © IngramPublishing p98, © Ivanchecko p69, © jonathandowney p102, © juniorbeep p11, © kumarworks p25, © LeggNet p70, © mikdam p49, © Neustockimages p116, © nicolesy p78, © olgaecat p8, © Pete Fleming p26, © phakimata p92, © PIKSEL p20, © pringletta p57, © Roberto A Sanchez p89, © RobLopshire p85, © schmidttty p132, © SciePro p109, © scottjay p66, © Sheryl Yazolino Griffin p39, © Thomas_EyeDesign p35, © tirc83 p64, © tomczykbartek p87, © VYCHEGZHANINA p44, © Yuri_Arcurs p48, © ZTS p45; **Jenni Lenard:** pp25, 120, 140; **JML:** p6; **Lars Carlsson (Makeup-FX.com):** pp119, 128; **Lash Perfect:** p130; **Mediscan:** p18; **Melissa Jenkins (www.melissajenkinsphotography.com):** p16; **Mundo:** pp33, 60; **Nail Delights (www.naildelights.com):** p131; **Nailtiques:** p88; **naturasun:** p9; **NSI (UK) Ltd. www.nsinails.co.uk:** p58, 130; **Oli Jones:** p81; **OPI for Scratch Magazine:** p128; **Orly:** p10; **Palms Extra:** p36; **Pasha Hammam by Hammam Couture:** pp44, 55, 58; **Professionails:** p60; **Sanrizz Education:** pp7, 7, 15, 15, 19, 21, 25, 26, 31, 32, 34, 40, 58, 64, 65, 66, 69, 71, 75, 75, 77, 79, 81, 91, 93, 97, 105, 105, 106, 110, 111, 114, 114, 114, 115, 117, 118, 120, 121, 124, 135, 136; **Science Photo Library:** p137; **Shutterstock:** © dpaint p54; **Spa Find Skincare:** p103; **St Tropez:** pp27, 34, 52, 87, 126; **Stephenson College:** pp19, 72, 93; **Sterex:** p119; **Studex:** p44; **Su-do:** p31; **The Airbrush Co Ltd.:** p91; **The British Association of Skin Camouflage:** p66; **The Edge Nail & Beauty:** pp6, 6, 9, 14, 14, 30, 57, 60, 81, 98; **The London College of Beauty Therapy:** p107; **The Sanctuary:** p37, 68; **The Training Company:** p115; **Tisserand (www.tisserand.com):** pp10, 17, 22, 23, 27, 42, 43, 50, 51, 62, 63, 63, 68, 73, 82, 84, 86, 86, 95, 96, 97, 98, 98, 100, 107, 117, 117, 119, 129, 129; **Tylo:** p127; **Walsall College:** p131; **Wella:** p114; **Workwear world:** p104; **Wow Factor:** p137; **www.sarahbmakeup.co.uk:** p93; **www.therapyessentials.co.uk:** p17; **www.ukvajazzled.co.uk:** p9.

INTRODUCTION –
HOW TO USE THIS BOOK

The City & Guilds A–Z contains the words you need to know if you're studying at Level 1, 2 or 3, or if you're a qualified beauty therapist or nail technician. So if you haven't heard of a technical word before or need to refresh your memory, look it up in here.

Each word is followed by a phonetic respelling, so you know exactly how to pronounce it, as well as the actual definition, so you know exactly what it means.

Spa

Spa – SPAH – The true meaning is a place that has naturally occurring mineral waters, such as Bath Spa or Leamington Spa in the UK. These are often hot when they come out through the earth.

Spa bath – SPAH BAHTH – This is often referred to as a jacuzzi or whirlpool. It has either circulating water or water forced through pipes to create a relaxing, bubbling effect.

Spa therapist – SPAH THERR-uh-pist – A therapist who specialises in spa treatments such as hydrotherapy and body wraps.

Special effects make-up – SPESH-uhl i-FEKTS MAYK-up – The creation of a look including wounds and injuries.

Specialist salons – SPESH-uh-list SAH-lo(ng)z or suh-LO(ng)z – Salons that specialise in certain services, for example male skin care, make-up for special occasions, etc.

Specialist skin care products – SPESH-uh-list SKIN KAIR PROD-uhkts – These are used to target specific skin improvement and include eye gels/creams, neck creams and lip products.

Sphenoid – SFEE-noyd – One bone forming the back of the eye sockets.

Spider naevi – SPIY-duh NEE-viy – This is usually a central small blood spot with thread veins, which radiates outwards.

Spillage – SPIL-ij – A product or substance that is dropped or leaked onto the floor.

Spine – SPIYN – The spine is made up of seven cervical bones, 12 thoracic bones, five lumbar bones, five bones fused together to make up the sacrum and four bones fused together to make up the coccyx.

The word

The phonetic respelling

The definition

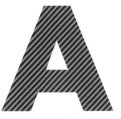

Abbreviation – uh-bree-vee-AY-shuhn – A shortened form of a word or phrase, normally used when making appointments, eg m/c (manicure), 1/2 LW (half leg wax), IHM (Indian Head Massage) and m/up (make-up).

Abdomen – AB-duh-muhn – The tummy area of the body.

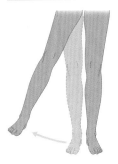

Abduction – uhb-DUK-shuhn – Anatomical term which means to take away from the midline, ie lifting the leg away from the body and out to the side.

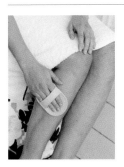

Abrasive mitts – uh-BRAY-siv MITS – A rough surface mitt used to remove fine hair and exfoliate the skin.

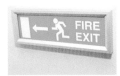

Abrasives – uh-BRAY-sivz – The term used to describe nail files and buffers.

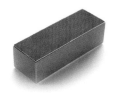

Access and egress – AK-sess uhnd EE-gress – All the routes into and out of the workplace. All corridors, doorways, steps and emergency exits, etc must be kept free from obstructions and well maintained.

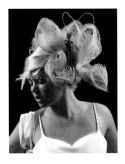

Accessory – uhk-SESS-uh-ree – An item, such as a fascinator, feathers or clips, used to complement a finished look.

Accident book – AK-sid-uhnt BUUK – A book in the workplace where accidents are recorded; this is a requirement of health and safety law.

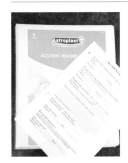

Accident form – AK-sid-uhnt FORM – A report to be recorded following any accident in the workplace.

Accutane – AK-yoo-tayn – An oral medication used for the treatment of severe acne. A side effect is thinned and sensitised skin, so is a contra-indication to micro-dermabrasion.

Acetone – ASS-i-tohn – A colourless liquid used in some nail varnish removers and for the removal of enhancements. Commonly known as tip remover.

Acid – ASS-id – The term used for a substance that is less than pH 7. These substances are commonly found in exfoliating products.

Acid mantle – ASS-id MANTL – The acid film on the skin which gives protection to the skin's surface.

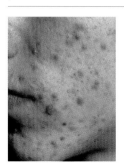

Acne vulgaris – AK-nee vul-GAH-ris – A skin condition where there is an increase in the production of sebum, causing congestion and inflammation.

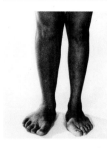

Acromegaly endocrine disorder – ak-roh-MEG-uh-lee END-oh-kriyn diss-OR-duh – A disorder caused by oversecretion of the pituitary gland. It can be identified by enlarged bones of the body, and is particularly noticeable in an enlarged head, feet and hands.

Acrylates – AK-ri-layts or AK-ri-luhts – The family of chemicals from which nail enhancements are created.

Acrylic – uh-KRIL-ik – A type of plastic. All nail enhancements are acrylic and made of polymers.

Acrylic-based paints – uh-KRIL-ik BAYSST PAYNTS – These contain water but have a high concentration of acrylic and high colour definition.

Actin – AK-tin – A protein found in muscles that is involved in muscle contraction.

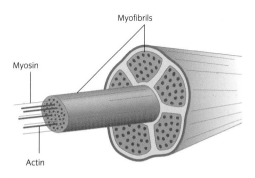

Myofibrils

Myosin

Actin

Action plan – AK-shuhn PLAN – Individuals can set personal goals that need to be achieved within a given timescale.

Activator – AK-ti-vay-tuh – This liquid speeds up the polymerisation process for a cyanoacrylate resin and is used within the wrap system.

Active electrode – AK-tiv i-LEK-trohd – Sometimes referred to as a working electrode, this is used in facial or body electrical treatments. The electrode is used on the skin and the current flows through.

Active listening – AK-tiv LISS-ning – Using techniques to show that you are paying close attention to what is being said by a client or colleague. For example, using eye contact, or repeating back what the person has said, to confirm understanding.

Acute dermatitis – uh-KYOOT dur-muh-TIY-tiss – Caused by exposure to an irritant and occurs almost immediately.

Acute toxicity – uh-KYOOT tok-SISS-it-ee – Essential oils being taken orally, or excessive use of essential oils on the skin, could lead to liver and kidney damage.

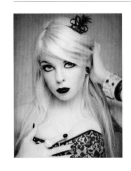

Additional media – uh-DISH-uhn-uhl MEE-dee-uh – These could be clothes, make-up, jewellery, props – in fact, anything you use to support your design.

Additional services or products – uh-DISH-uhn-uhl SUR-viss-iz or PROD-uhkts – The additional services of which clients may not be aware, such as make-up services and the products that your salon stocks.

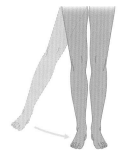

Adduction – uh-DUK-shuhn – Anatomical term which means to bring towards the midline, ie bringing the leg back towards the body.

Adductor brevis, longus and magnus – uh-DUK-tuh BREV-iss, LONG-giss uhnd MAG-nuhss – Three muscles on the inner side of the upper thigh. They adduct, rotate and flex the thigh.

Adhesive – uhd-HEE-siv – A cyanoacrylate adhesive that is safe to use on the skin and bonds the tip to the nail. It's often incorrectly called glue.

Adipose tissue – AD-i-pohz TISH-yoo – The layer of fat cells which lies beneath the dermis, otherwise known as the subcutaneous layer.

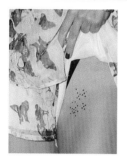

Adornments – uh-DORN-muhnts – Usually in the form of diamanté crystals, these are available as pre-made patterns, such as hearts and dolphins, on an adhesive backing, or as individual stones, which are applied following intimate waxing.

Adrenaline – uh-DREN-uh-lin – A hormone which prepares the body for fight or flight. It raises the blood sugar level and stimulates the nervous system.

Adverse reaction – AD-vurss ree-AK-shuhn – When a client has a negative reaction to a skin test carried out prior to any treatment.

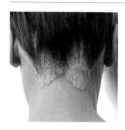

Adverse skin, scalp and hair conditions – AD-vurss SKIN, SKALP uhnd HAIR kuhn-DISH-uhnz – Conditions that can stop, limit or restrict a service or treatment. Examples include impetigo, scars, moles, psoriasis and alopecia.

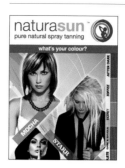

naturasun™
pure natural spray tanning
what's your colour?

Advertising – AD-vuh-tiyz-ing – Forms of communication with the purpose of persuading the client to buy.

Advice – uhd-VIYSS – Knowledge given to the client after the treatment so that they can continue its benefits.

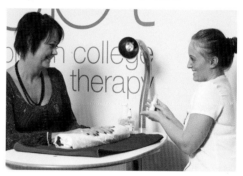

Advice on employment issues – uhd-VIYSS on im-PLOY-muhnt ISH-ooz – You can seek advice from the Citizens Advice Bureau, trade unions, a private solicitor, or a training provider (if under a government funded training scheme).

Aerobic exercise – air-ROH-bik EKS-uh-siyz – Exercise that increases the body's need for oxygen in order to improve respiratory and circulatory functions. It burns fat and increases the heart rate.

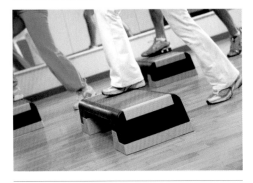

Affusion shower – uh-FYOO-zhuhn SHOW-uh – A treatment where the client lies on a couch while water from micro jets above is applied. It is sometimes called a rain shower.

Aftercare – AHF-tuh-KAIR – Advice given to the client following treatment.

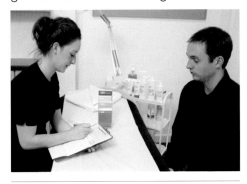

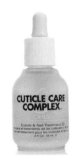

Aftercare products – AHF-tuh-KAIR PROD-uhkts – Products such as cuticle oils, moisturisers and cleansers that prolong the benefits of the treatment after the client has left the salon.

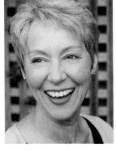

Age group – AYJ groop – An age range which describes a person, eg post-16, post-31 and post-50. You might need to consider a client's age sometimes, for example if creating a make-up look.

Ageing skin – AYJ-ing SKIN – Skin that shows signs of ageing. It can be identified by dryness, wrinkles, poor elasticity or weakened muscle tone, and can be accelerated by many factors (the most common being sunlight).

AHA (Alpha hydroxy acids) – AY-AICH-AY -- AL-fuh hiy-DROK-see ASS-idz – Chemical substances commonly found in facial products that exfoliate the skin. The most common AHA is glycolic acid, which comes from sugar cane.

AIDS (Acquired Immunodeficiency Syndrome) – AYDZ -- uh-KWIY-uhd i-MYOO-noh-di-FISH-uhn-see SIN-drohm – AIDS develops as a result of being infected with the HIV virus. It reduces the body's ability to fight infection.

Air blower – AIR BLOH-uh – A gentle puffer used in the application of single eyelash extensions to speed the drying process of the adhesive bonding agent.

Air hose – AIR hohz – The hose that travels from the compressor to the airbrush.

Air pressure – AIR PRESH-uh – The pressure used to push the air through the airbrush.

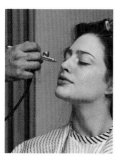

Airbrushing (for make-up) – AIR-BRUSH-ing – In make-up this means using a compressor to spray a fine mist of product onto a surface. Airbrush tools consist of a trigger, compressor and reservoir.

Airbrushing (for nail art) – AIR-BRUSH-ing – A nail art technique. A brush is attached to a compressor by a hose and held in the hand. Air is mixed with paint before being forced out to create a coloured spray.

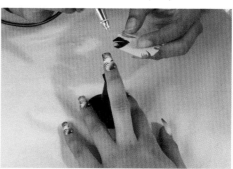

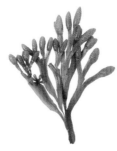

Algae – AL-jee or AL-jiy or AL-gee or AL-giy – A detoxifying seaweed containing therapeutic minerals. It is often found in body wraps and is sometimes added to the water in a hydrotherapy bath.

Alkaline – AL-kuh-liyn – The term used for a substance that is more than pH 7. These substances are commonly found in facial galvanic products.

Allergen – AL-uh-juhn – A substance that causes your immune system to react abnormally.

Allergic reaction – uh-LUR-jik ree-AK-shuhn – Appears in the form of irritation, discomfort, itching and reddening.

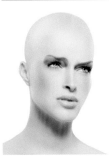

Alopecia – al-uh-PEE-shuh – This is the term used for hair loss, whether it is a small bald patch or total hair loss over the whole body. It usually results from shock, trauma, illness or prolonged stress.

Alternating current – OL-tuh-nay-ting KUH-ruhnt – The type of current that comes through the mains socket and reverses backwards and forwards.

Amenorrhoea – ay-men-uh-REE-uh – Absence of the menstrual cycle. This may be due to drastic weight loss or endocrine disorders.

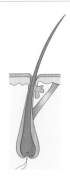

Anagen hair – AN-uh-juhn HAIR – The active stage of hair growth, where the hair is still attached to its blood supply. This is the best stage for successful epilation.

Anaphoresis – an-uh-fuh-REE-siss – The use of a negative galvanic current to help dilate small, tight follicles before treatment, making insertion easier.

Anaphylactic shock – AN-uh-fi-LAK-tik SHOK – An extreme allergic reaction which can be fatal.

Androgens – AN-druh-juhnz – Hormones that can cause excess hair growth in women. Also known as hirsutism.

Anion – AN-iy-uhn – A negatively charged ion that moves to the anode.

Anode – AN-ohd – An electrode that is positively charged on the machine. It can be identified by the + sign.

Antagonist – an-TAG-uh-nist – When one muscle contracts the opposite muscle works in the opposite way, this is referred to as antagonist. An example is when the biceps contract, creating a biceps curl.

Anterior – an-TEER-ee-uh – The front surface or front of the body.

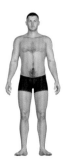

Anti-ageing – an-tee-AYJ-ing – Products or treatments that are designed to protect the skin from the ageing process or slow it down.

Antibacterial – an-tee-bak-TEER-ee-uhl – A substance that prevents or stops the growth of bacteria.

Antiperspirant – an-tee-PURSS-puh-ruhnt – Used to reduce underarm perspiration.

Antiseptic – an-tee-SEP-tik – A substance that will reduce the growth of micro-organisms that cause diseases.

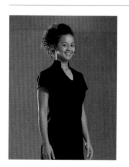

Apocrine glands – AP-uh-kriyn or AP-uh-krin or AP-uh-kreen GLANDZ – Sweat glands that are found on the hairy areas, eg under the arms and pubic regions. They produce sweat which also contains a fatty substance.

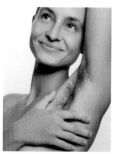

Appearance – uh-PEER-ruhnss – How you present yourself in the salon environment.

Appendicular skeleton – ap-uhn-DIK-yuh-luh SKEL-it-uhn – Made up of the shoulder girdle, pelvic girdle, legs and arms.

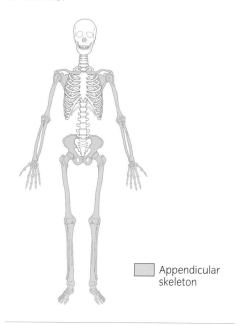

Appendicular skeleton

Application tools – ap-li-KAY-shuhn TOOLZ – Tools used during a treatment, eg brushes, sponges and velour puffs used in camouflage make-up.

Appointment – uh-POYNT-muhnt – A pre-arranged service booked for a scheduled day and time.

Appointment details – uh-POYNT-muhnt DEE-taylz – Recorded information that relates to the appointment, eg date, time, service, expected service duration and name of the beauty therapist.

Appointment system – uh-POYNT-muhnt SISS-tuhm – A method used for recording client appointment bookings – it could be on a computer or in a book.

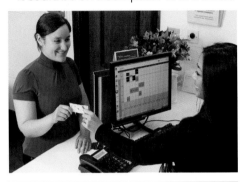

Appraisal – uh-PRAY-zuhl – A regular review of your progress that will be done by your line manager. This will help you to know what you're doing well and where your development needs are.

Appropriate language – uh-PROHP-ree-uht LANG-gwij – Suitable language that helps you to communicate effectively with clients. You should not use words that are too technical. Appropriate language is always clear, polite and friendly.

Aroma-stone – uh-ROH-muh-STOHN – A small electrical heated appliance used to warm essential oils so they're dispersed into the air.

Arrector pili muscle – uh-REK-tuh PILL-ee MUSS-uhl – A tiny muscle attached to the hair follicle. When it contracts, it causes the hair to stand on end. This happens when the body is cold and the raised hairs trap air, insulating and warming the body.

Arteriole – ah-TEER-ree-ohl – A tiny artery which is bigger than a capillary.

Artery – AH-tuh-ree – Transports mainly oxygenated blood to the cells and tissues.

Arthritis – ahth-RY-tiss – A condition that affects the joints of the body and causes inflammation, pain and difficulty moving.

Artificial lash remover – ah-ti-FISH-uhl LASH ri-MOO-vuh – A type of solvent that is used to remove lash adhesive.

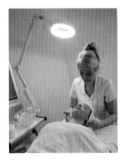

Artificial light – ah-ti-FISH-uhl LIYT – Light that is not sunlight, for example the light from a magnifying lamp.

Artificial nail structure – ah-ti-FISH-uhl NAYL STRUK-chuh – A structure that is applied on top of the natural nail.

Aseptic – ay-SEP-tik – A bacteria-free area; a therapist should always try to work in an area like this. This can be achieved by thorough cleaning, wearing gloves, sterilising equipment and disposing of waste properly.

Assembly point – uh-SEM-blee POYNT – The designated meeting point in the event of an emergency evacuation.

Assessment – uh-SESS-muhnt – An evaluation or judgement of a candidate's work performance. There are several methods of assessment, eg oral questions, written questions, witness testimonies, and assessment of prior learning and/or experience.

Assignment – uh-SIYN-muhnt – A set task or practical activity.

Asthma – AS-muh or AS-thmuh – A disorder of the respiratory system which causes the airways to narrow, leaving the person breathless and wheezy.

Astringent – uh-STRIN-juhnt – A strong product used to tone the skin; it often has a drying effect on the skin.

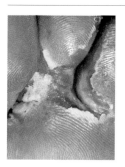

Athlete's foot – ATH-leets FUUT – A fungal infection known as tinea pedis. The skin between the toes becomes moist and white, and is often itchy and inflamed.

Atrophic scar – uh-TROF-ik SKAH or uh-TROH-fik SKAH – This type of scar is depressed and indented, causing a valley or hole in the skin.

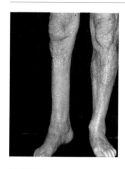

Atrophy – AT-ruh-fee – Muscle wastage where the muscle lacks tone and strength. It often occurs after an injury, eg when wearing a plaster cast.

Axillary – ak-SIL-uh-ree – Lymph nodes in the underarm.

Audio sonic – OR-dee-oh SON-ik – A hand-held device utilising sound waves, which penetrate the skin to a depth of 2.5 inches and which travel and vibrate along the inside of the muscle sheath.

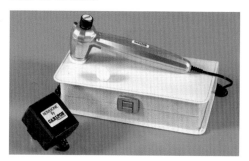

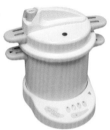

Autoclave

– OR-toh-klayv – A device for sterilising beauty and nail metal tools in very hot pressurised steam.

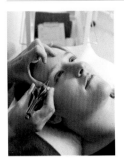

Automatic tweezers – or-tuh-MAT-ik TWEE-zuhz – These are spring-loaded – use with care – and are used to remove a bulk of hair.

Autonomic nervous system –

or-tuh-NOM-ik NUR-vuhss SISS-tuhm – Controls the involuntary activities of smooth and cardiac muscle, as well as the glands. It consists of both sympathetic and parasympathetic.

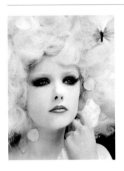

Avant-garde

– AV-o(ng)-GAHD – A style, look or image that is ahead of the times, usually worn or produced by the leaders of fashion, before it becomes fashionable.

Axial skeleton – AKS-ee-uhl SKEL-it-uhn – Made up of the skull, spine (vertebral column), ribs and sternum.

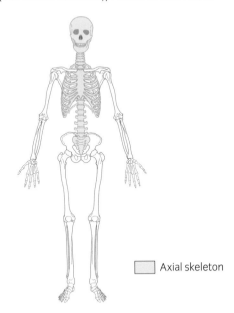

☐ Axial skeleton

Ayurveda – iy-uh-VAY-duh or iy-uh-VEE-duh – A healing system that comes from a sacred Hindu text, describing how the mind, body and spirit should be in harmony to improve the heath and wellbeing of the person.

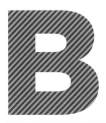

Basalt stone – BASS-orlt STOHN – A black volcanic rock that absorbs and retains heat well. Its penetrative warmth helps to release deep muscular tension and congestion, and improves the general circulation.

Back bubbling – BAK BUB-uh-ling – Blocking the nozzle of the airbrush to redirect the flow of air back to the cup. This can aid cleaning or colour mixing.

Back, sack and crack – BAK SAK uhnd KRAK – A treatment where hair is removed from the lower back, buttocks and scrotum.

Bacteria – bak-TEER-ee-uh – Single-celled micro-organism. It can be both disease causing (pathogenic) or non-disease causing (non-pathogenic).

Bad breath – BAD BRETH – Noticeably unpleasant odours exhaled in breathing – another term for this is halitosis.

Basal cell carcinoma – BAY-suhl SEL kah-si-NOH-muh – A form of skin cancer which grows slowly and has the appearance of a skin growth that does not heal and bleeds frequently.

Basal metabolic rate – BAY-suhl met-uh-BOL-ik RAYT – A measure of calories burned while at rest.

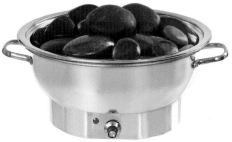

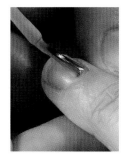

Base coat – BAYSS koht – This is applied before the coloured nail varnish to smooth the nail, cut down on staining and to help prevent the varnish from chipping.

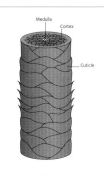

Basic structure of the hair – BAYSS-ik STRUK-chuh uhv dhuh HAIR – The basic structure of the hair is made up of the cuticle, cortex and medulla.

Basic structure of the nail – BAYSS-ik STRUK-chuh uhv dhuh NAYL – The basic structure of the nail is made up of the nail plate, nail wall, cuticle and free edge.

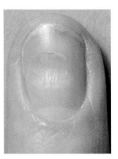

Beau's lines
– BOHZ liynz – Lines or deep grooves that run across the nail plate. May be caused by an injury to the nail.

Beauty therapist – BYOO-tee THERR-uh-pist – A person who is qualified to carry out a variety of treatments within a beauty salon or spa, for example facial cleansing or a body massage.

Beauty-related terminology – BYOO-tee ri-LAYT-id tur-min-OL-uh-jee – A specialised vocabulary used within the beauty-related industries.

Behaviour – bi-HAYV-ee-uh – How you behave includes following instructions, working co-operatively with others and following salon requirements.

Behavioural expectations – bi-HAYV-ee-uh-ruhl ek-spek-TAY-shuhnz – You will be expected to work co-operatively with others, and following salon requirements.

Benefits – BEN-uh-fits – These describe why the client would want to buy your products or services. For example, a product's benefit may be that it improves skin condition.

Benefits of effective team working – BEN-uh-fits uhv i-FEK-tive TEEM WUR-king – The benefits include: client satisfaction, personal and team achievement, positive salon reputation, repeat business, staff motivation and morale, and harmony within the working environment.

BHAs (Beta-hydroxy acids) – BEE-tuh hiy-DROKS-ee ASS-idz -- BEE AICH AYZ – Specifically describes salicylic acid, which is derived from plants. They are used for exfoliating treatments and are more gentle than AHAs.

Biceps – BIY-seps – Anterior upper arm muscle that flexes the forearm.

Biceps femoris – BIY-seps FEM-uh-riss – One of the muscles that forms the hamstrings. It runs from the pelvis, down the back of the leg to the tibia and extends the hip and flexes the knee.

Bikini shaping – bi-KEE-nee SHAY-ping – This involves trimming and waxing the pubic hair into shapes such as a star or a heart, either using a template or freehand.

Blend method – BLEND METH-uhd – A combination of direct galvanic current and alternating high frequency current (diathermy) passing down the same needle. This has the efficiency of galvanic electrolysis, with a faster speed. It can result in a more effective, less painful treatment.

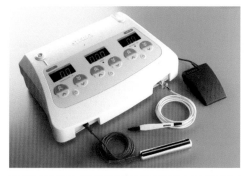

Blending – BLEN-ding – A technique used in make-up which mixes two colours together.

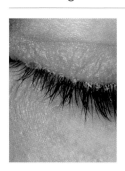

Blepharitis – blef-uh-RIY-tiss – Inflammation of the eyelid or eyelid rims. The eyes feel red, irritated and itchy. Dandruff-like crusts can appear on the eyelashes.

Blocked pore – BLOKT POR – A build-up of sebum in the follicle opening. They are usually creamy coloured. If the sebum oxidises with the air and turns black they are then referred to as comedones.

Blood capillary – BLUD kuh-PIL-uh-ree – The smallest blood vessel that is one cell thick. It allows the exchange of various substances, such as oxygen and nutrients into the cells, and carbon dioxide and waste out of the cells.

Blood pressure – BLUD PRESH-uh – The force of pressure on the arteries due to the contraction of the left ventricle. The maximum pressure is called Systolic – this is when the heart contracts. The minimum pressure is called Diastolic – this is when the heart relaxes.

Blood pulse – BLUD PULSS – This is felt in the arteries that are close to the surface of the skin. It indicates the pumping action of the heart.

Blood vessels – BLUD VESS-uhlz – Carry blood around the body.

Blushers – BLUSH-uhz – These come in a variety of different forms, including creams, powders and liquids, and are used to enhance the cheekbones.

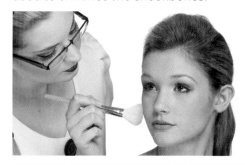

Body analysis – BOD-ee uh-NAL-uh-siss – A careful assessment of the body to determine, amongst other things, its shape, type and condition, posture and height to weight ratio, taking into account contributory factors.

Body areas – BOD-ee AIR-ee-uhz – The areas that can be worked on, such as the lower legs, arms, shoulders or face.

Body galvanic – BOD-ee gal-VAN-ik – This uses the principle of iontophoresis to introduce beneficial substances into the skin. In the case of body treatments the substance will usually be diuretic, to help reduce the appearance of cellulite.

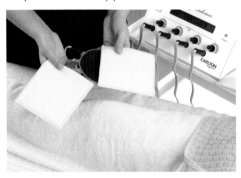

Body image – BOD-ee IM-ij – How a person views his or her own body. This may be accurate, but may also be a flawed perception.

Body language – BOD-ee LANG-gwij – A way of communicating to our clients or colleagues using our bodies but not using speech.

Body mass index (BMI) – BOD-ee MASS IN-deks -- BEE-EM-IY – An indicator of whether a client's weight is appropriate to their height. This is calculated by dividing weight by height. A normal BMI is between 20 and 25.

Body micro-current – BOD-ee MY-kroh KURR-uhnt – An electrical treatment used in various ways to lift and firm body contours.

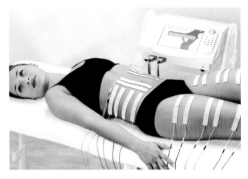

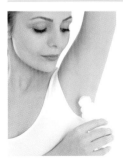

Body odour – BOD-ee OH-duh – Body odour, sometimes abbreviated as B.O., is the smell of bacteria growing on the body. The bacteria multiply rapidly in the presence of sweat, but sweat itself is almost completely odourless to humans.

Body wrap

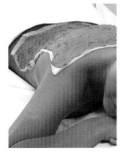

– BOD-ee RAP – A treatment where a specific product is applied to the body. The body is then wrapped in bandages, plastic sheets or thermal blankets to achieve effects including stimulation of the circulation, detoxification and relaxation.

Boils (also known as furuncles)

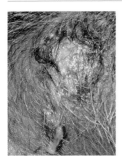

– BOYLZ -- FYOO-runklz – Bacterial infection around the base of a hair follicle. The symptoms include swelling, redness, pain and pus.

Bollywood – BOL-ee-wuud – Intimate waxing where the skin is subsequently decorated by application of a henna pattern.

Bone structure of the face – BOHN STRUK-chuh uhv dhuh FAYSS – The bones of the face include the mandible, maxillae, zygomatic and frontal.

Bones of the head and neck – BOHNZ uhv dhuh HED uhnd NEK – The bones in the head are the occipital, frontal, parietal, temporal, sphenoid and ethmoid; the bones in the neck are the cervical vertebrae.

Botox – BOH-toks – Botox is one brand of botulinum toxin type A. This is a neurotoxin that blocks nerve signals to muscles, stopping or limiting their movement.

Bottom feed – BOT-uhm FEED – Commonly used for spray tanning. A large plastic cup is placed underneath the airbrush to hold the fluid.

Boyzilian – boy-ZIL-ee-uhn – Similar to a female Brazilian, male Brazilian waxing is characterised by a small strip of hair above the penis.

Brachio radialis – BRAY-kee-oh ray-dee-AL-iss – Muscle between the upper arm and forearm. It flexes the forearm.

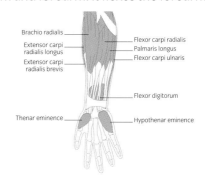

Brachio radialis
Extensor carpi radialis longus
Extensor carpi radialis brevis
Thenar eminence
Flexor carpi radialis
Palmaris longus
Flexor carpi ulnaris
Flexor digitorum
Hypothenar eminence

Brazilian – bruh-ZIL-ee-uhn – Hair is removed from the pubic area apart from a strip approximately 2.5 cm wide up and over the pubic mound.

Breach of security – BREECH uhv suh-KYOO-uh-ri-tee – When someone gets in somewhere they shouldn't have been able to, for example if the salon is broken into at night.

Breathing zone – BREEDH-ing ZOHN – The area surrounding the nail technician's air supply.

Brittle nails – BRITL NAYLZ – Nails that snap easily. This can be caused by hands being constantly in water and chemicals.

Broad spectrum protection – BROHD SPEK-truhm pruh-TEK-shuhn – Protects against UVA/B and environmental damage.

Bruising – BROO-zing – A trauma caused to the skin when it has suffered some kind of blow.

Buccal – BUK-uhl – Lymph nodes found either side of the mouth.

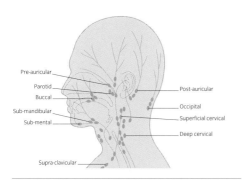

Pre-auricular
Parotid
Buccal
Sub-mandibular
Sub-mental
Post-auricular
Occipital
Superficial cervical
Deep cervical
Supra-clavicular

Buccinator – BUK-sin-ay-tuh – Muscle that lies below the risorius.

Budget – BUJ-it – The amount of money available to spend on a project.

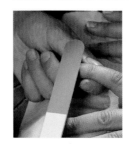

Buffing – BUF-ing – A technique used to create a shine on the nail.

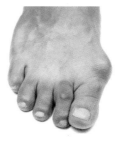

Bunion – BUN-yuhn – Also known as hallux valgus, this is a thickening of the bone or tissue around the joint at the base of the big toe. This causes the toe to turn inwards, and the joint swells and feels tender.

Business – BIZ-niss – An organisation engaged in the sale of goods and/or services.

Buying signal – BIY-ing SIG-nuhl – A comment from a client, which indicates that they are thinking about buying your product or service. The most common buying signal is the question: 'How much is it?'. Others are questions or comments such as: 'What sizes does it come in?'. Surprisingly, 'It's too expensive' or 'I already have a similar product at home' are also buying signals!

By-laws – BIY-lohz – Local laws passed from a higher authority and can vary from place to place. Contact your local HSE for more information about your area's by-laws.

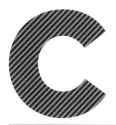

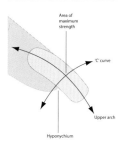

'C' curve – SEE-kurv – The natural curve of the nail from side wall to side wall. You need to look down the finger from the end to see the 'C' curve.

Calamine – KAL-uh-miyn or KAL-uh-min – A fine mineral powder used in face masks. It is calming and soothing, and is very good for irritated, sensitive skins.

Calcaneus – kal-KAY-nee-uhss – More commonly known as the heel bone.

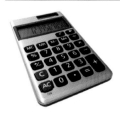

Calculate – KALK-yoo-layt – This is when you do some maths, eg adding up the client's bill for all the services, or when you need to work out mixing ratios.

Caldarium – kal-DAIR-ree-uhm – The hottest steam room where herbal essences may be used to create a pleasant, perfumed steam.

Californian – kal-i-FORN-ee-uhn – Intimate waxing where the remaining hair is tinted.

Callous – KAL-uhs – Commonly found on the heel of the foot. Thick, yellowish, hardened skin that can be cracked and may even bleed.

Camouflage products – KAM-uh-flahzh PROD-uhkts – Products used during a camouflage application, eg camouflage cream, camouflage powders and setting powders.

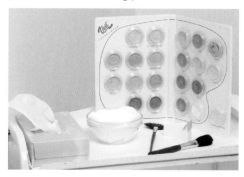

Carbide bits – KAH-biyd BITS – The long-lasting bits on the electric file (or e-file) that shave the surface of the overlay with a scooping action, producing large dust particles.

Career opportunities – kuh-REER op-uh-TYOON-it-eez – The roles and places in which you may work once you are qualified.

Carpals – KAH-puhlz – Eight small bones that form the wrist and each have a separate name.

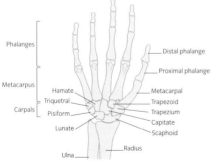

Carrier oils – KARR-eer OYLZ – Oily plant base used to dilute essential oils for use on the skin.

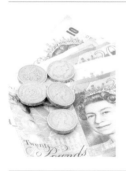

Cash – KASH – Banknotes and coins.

Cash equivalent – KASH i-KWIV-uh-luhnt – When a client pays with a voucher or a points system.

Cash flow forecast – KASH FLOH FOR-kahst – An estimate of when and how much money will be received and paid out of a business.

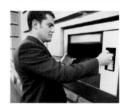

Cashpoint – KASH-poynt – Where you insert your debit/credit card and enter your PIN to obtain cash.

Cashing up – KASH-ing uhp – At the end of a day's business, the till is counted to see if the takings are accurate for the day.

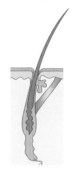

Catagen hair – KAT-uh-jen HAIR – The stage in the hair growth cycle where the hair begins to detach from the dermal papilla and receives its nutrients from the follicle wall.

Catalyst – KAT-uh-list – An additive that works with the initiator and controls the speed of the chemical reaction.

Cataphoresis – kat-uh-fuh-REE-siss – The use of a positive galvanic current commonly used after epilation to help constrict follicles, reduce redness and rebalance the acid mantle, making bacterial infection less likely.

Cathode – KATH-ohd – An electrode that is negatively charged on the machine. It is identified by the – sign.

Cation – KAT-iy-uhn – A positively charged ion that moves to the cathode.

Catwalk show – KAT-work SHOH – N.B. 'walk' rhymes with 'fork' – Usually performed on a runway, it features models who are showcasing a designer's clothes or new collections.

Cauterise – KOR-tuh-riyz – A term used in electrical epilation to refer to destroying the tissue, dermal papilla and hair follicle by the direct application of heat at a high temperature.

Cell mitosis – SEL miy-TOH-siss – Cell division that is also referred to as cell metabolism and cellular renewal.

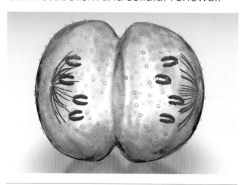

Cellulite – SEL-yuh-liyt – Congested tissue with a dimply 'orange peel' appearance. It is usually cold to the touch and commonly found on the thighs and buttocks.

Central nervous system – SEN-truhl NUR-vuhss SISS-tuhm – Made up of the brain and spinal cord.

Certificate of registration – suh-TIF-ik-uht uhv rej-iss-TRAY-shuhn – This is awarded when salon premises have been successfully inspected to ensure that they are complying with local by-laws in relation to cosmetic piercing.

Cervical vertebrae – SURV-ikl VUR-tuh-bray/VUR-tuh-bree – Seven discs forming the top part of the spine. The first, the 'atlas', supports the skull and the second, the 'axis', rotates the skull.

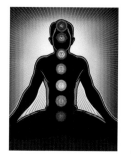

Chakras – CHAK-ruhz or CHUK-ruhz – Energy centres that do not have a physical form and are a way of describing energies and energy flow. They are the focal points for restoring balance to the body. There are seven major Chakras – Indian head massage refers to the three higher Chakras.

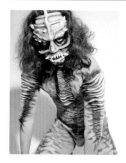

Character make-up – KARR-ak-tuh MAYK-up – Changing a subject's physical appearance to suit the requirements of a script or part to be played. This may include changes in age, emphasis of particular facial features and so on.

Cheek products – CHEEK PROD-uhkts – Cosmetics applied to cheeks to add colour and emphasise facial contours.

Chemical skin peeling – KEM-ikl SKIN PEE-ling – This treatment involves the application of a chemical solution to the skin.

Chemotherapy – KEE-moh-THERR-uh-pee – A course of drug treatments used to kill cancerous cells.

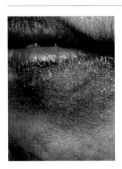

Cheque – CHEK – A form of payment for a service; cheques must be accompanied by a cheque guarantee card.

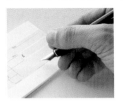

Chloasma/ melasma – kloh-AZ-muh/muh-LAZ-muh – A hyper-pigmentation disorder resulting in areas of increased pigmentation. Darker patches of skin compared to other areas will be visible.

Chlorhexidine acetate – klor-HEKS-i-diyn ASS-it-ayt – A medical antiseptic with bactericidal properties.

Cholesterol – kuh-LESS-tuh-ruhl – A type of fat that is manufactured in the liver or intestines, but is also found in some of the foods of animal origin we eat.

Chronic dermatitis – KRON-ik dur-muh-TIY-tiss – Caused by overexposure to an irritant over a period of time, be it days, weeks, months or years.

Chronic toxicity – KRON-ik tok-SISS-it-ee – This is when an essential oil has been overused repeatedly over a period of time.

Circulation – surk-yuh-LAY-shuhn – The movement of substances around the body – oxygen and nutrient are transported to the cells, whereas carbon dioxide and waste are transported from the cells.

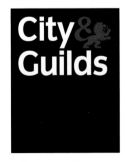

City & Guilds – SIT-ee uhnd GILDZ – The leading awarding body in hairdressing and beauty therapy qualifications. City & Guilds offers qualifications over a range of industry sectors through colleges and training providers in many countries worldwide.

Clavicle – KLAV-ikl – More commonly known as the collarbone, it forms a joint with the scapulae and sternum.

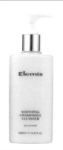

Cleanser – KLEN-zuh – A product that removes make-up, oil, dead skin cells, dirt and dust from the skin and pores.

Client – KLIY-uhnt – A person, sometimes referred to as customer, who visits the salon for treatments. It might also be a person who is commissioning a photo shoot. They may not always be present on the day, so you need to make sure you've designed exactly what they asked for.

Client care – KLIY-uhnt KAIR – Being able to treat the client with respect and professionalism at all times. Realising this is the key to your success.

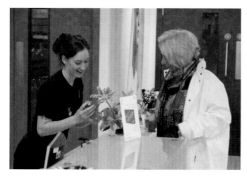

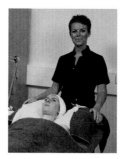

Client preparation – KLIY-uhnt prep-uh-RAY-shuhn – Preparing the client for the service by using towels to protect the client's clothes, covering their hair with a headband and positioning them comfortably.

Client records – KLIY-uhnt REK-ordz – Confidential records kept by the salon. They list the client's details such as address, contact number and treatment history.

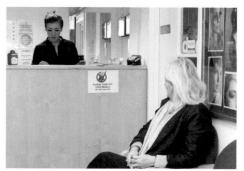

Client satisfaction – KLIY-uhnt sat-is-FAK-shuhn – When the client's expectations for the service have been met by the therapist.

Client specification or brief – KLIY-uhnt spess-if-i-KAY-shuhn or BREEF – A description of what the client is looking for, usually in written form.

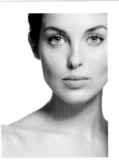

Client's features – KLIY-uhnts FEE-chuhz – Eyes, ears, cheekbones and other factors that are taken into consideration when producing a make-up look for the client.

Client's requirements – KLIY-uhnts ruh-KWIY-uh-muhnts – Any requests from the client; it may not always be possible to meet their needs, so a compromise may be needed.

Client's rights – KLIY-uhnts RIYTS – These are the client's rights to be protected as a consumer or purchaser of services and goods within your salon. Most of these rights come from laws, such as The Sale of Goods Act, The Supply of Goods and Services Act, The Consumer Protection Act and the Unfair Contract Terms Act. It's important to know what your client's rights are, in order to ensure that you comply with them.

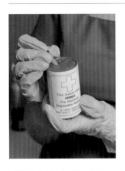

Clinical waste – KLIN-ikl WAYST – Waste that has been soiled with bodily fluids or skin tissue.

Closed questions – KLOHZD KWES-chuhnz – Questions that lead to yes and no answers, for example 'do your nails break easily?'.

Closing the sale – KLOH-zing dhuh SAYL – Gaining agreement from the client to buy.

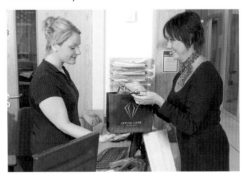

Club hair – KLUB HAIR – Refers to a hair in the catagen stage of hair growth. As the bulb has lost its shape, it detaches from the dermal papilla.

Co-operation – koh-op-uh-RAY-shuhn – Working together effectively to meet a common objective.

Coagulation – koh-ag-yuh-LAY-shuhn – A term used in electrical epilation to refer to destroying the tissue, dermal papilla and hair follicle by the direct application of heat that slowly heats the moist tissue.

Coconut oil – KOH-kuh-nut OYL – An oil often used in Indian head massage. This light, moisturising oil is derived from coconut and relieves inflammation.

Code of practice – KOHD uhv PRAK-tiss – Set rules of working, laid out by the industry or by the workplace itself.

Cold sore – KOHLD SOR – Also known as herpes simplex. Small, blister-like wounds that usually appear around the mouth. They are caused by the herpes simplex virus.

Cold stones – KOHLD STOHNZ – Stones which are cooled by placing them in ice or very cold water, and applied to the body in stone therapies. Marble stones are commonly used.

Collagen – KOL-uh-juhn – A protein that gives the skin strength and keeps it looking plump.

Colleagues – KOL-eegz – The people you work with.

Colour blending – KUH-luh BLEN-ding – Mixing two or more colours or products together to create a multi-coloured design. Can be used in body art, nail art or any make-up.

Colour fade – KUH-luh FAYD – An airbrushing technique, where an area of colour goes from dark to light and vice versa.

Colour spectrum – KUH-luh SPEK-truhm – Made up of the primary and secondary colours: red, orange, yellow, green, blue and violet.

Colour washing – KUH-luh WOSH-ing – Building a base of several thin coats of make-up.

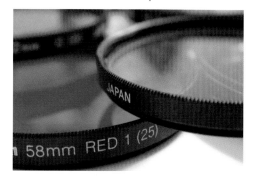

Colour wheel – KUH-luh WEEL – A visual representation of colours arranged into a circle or wheel that shows relationships between primary, secondary and complementary colours, etc.

P – Primary   T – Tertiary   S – Secondary

Coloured filters – KUH-luhd FIL-tuhz – These are used to change the mood of a photograph. It is important to understand the effect that these will have on the make-up.

Combustible – kuhm-BUST-uhbl – The tendency of something to react with oxygen and catch fire.

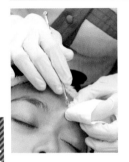

Comedone extractor – KOM-i-dohn ik-STRAK-tuh – A metal implement used to release comedones (also known as blackheads).

Comedone – KOM-i-dohn – PLURAL = **comedones** – KOM-i-dohnz – A blackhead – a plug of oxidised sebum in the follicle or pore opening that has turned black due to oxidisation with the air.

Commercial viability – kuh-MUR-shuhl viy-uh-BIL-it-ee – Making sure you don't spend too much time on tasks. If you take too long doing one thing, your salon loses money because you could be doing something else more valuable for the business. Remember that time is money and you're being paid to be efficient.

Commission – kuh-MISH-uhn – An incentive from your employer to encourage you to make recommendations and boost your monthly wage, as well as the salon's profits.

Communication – kuh-MYOO-ni-KAY-shuhn – The way we talk to others, ie the giving, receiving and reacting to information. This might be face-to-face, over the phone or through email.

Communication skills – kuh-MYOO-ni-KAY-shuhn SKILZ – The ability to pass on information accurately by listening carefully, and talking and writing clearly. You should be polite, friendly, helpful and respectful when communicating with clients.

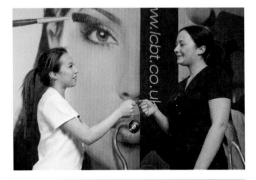

Compatibility tests – kuhm-pat-uh-BIL-it-ee tests – These tests are carried out to make sure the make-up base/foundation colours match the client's skin colouring.

Compensation – kom-pen-SAY-shuhn – A form of insurance that provides wage replacement and medical benefits to employees who have incurred work-related injuries.

Competition work – kom-puh-TISH-uhn WURK – Competing against others to achieve a common goal.

Complaint – kuhm-PLAYNT – When a client is not happy with a service; you need to remain calm and courteous at all times.

Complementary colours – kom-pluh-MEN-tree KUH-luhz – Colours that go together well.

Compound hair – KOM-pownd HAIR – A single follicle producing two or more hairs. It can also be referred to as a compound follicle.

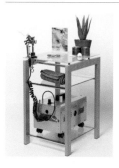

Compressor – kuhm-PRESS-uh – The equipment used as the source of air supply when airbrushing nail art or applying self-tanning products.

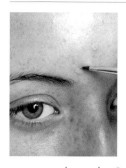

Concealer – kuhn-SEE-luh – A product used to cover any imperfections, usually applied before foundation. Common colours used include green and purple. Green neutralises red and purple helps to disguise dark circles.

Confidential information – kon-fi-DEN-shuhl in-fuh-MAY-shuhn – Private information that must not be passed on. It may include personal aspects of conversations with clients or colleagues, client details held on record cards, staff personal details or financial aspects of the business.

Confidentiality – kon-fi-den-shee-AL-it-ee – Keeping information/data private. It's important to keep clients' information confidential in order to ensure trust between yourself and your client.

Congenital abnormality – kuhn-JEN-it-uhl ab-nor-MAL-it-ee – This is a skin condition present since birth, eg port-wine stains.

Congenital hair growth – kuhn-JEN-it-uhl HAIR GROHTH – Excessive hairiness that is present from birth in some people. For example, it may appear as a very hairy mole or as a birthmark covered in hair. In extreme cases the whole body might be covered in thick terminal hair.

Conjunctiva – kon-junk-TIY-vuh – The outermost layer of the eye and the inner surface of the eyelids.

Conjunctivitis – kuhn-junk-ti-VIY-tiss – An inflammation of the conjunctiva, most commonly due to an allergic reaction or an infection.

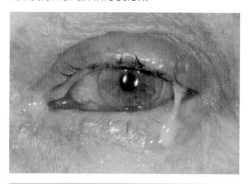

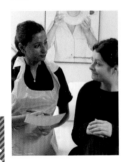

Consultation
– kon-sul-TAY-shuhn – Carried out before any beauty treatment begins. The therapist must assess the client's needs using different techniques, eg questioning and touch.

Consultation techniques – kon-sul-TAY-shuhn tek-NEEKS – Methods of finding out relevant information from your client so you can plan and perform a nail service.

Consumables – kuhn-SYOOM-uhblz – An item which cannot be reused, eg a cotton bud.

Consumer – kuhn-SYOO-muh – The client buying the treatment, service or product.

Consumer and retail legislation – kuhn-SYOO-muh uhnd REE-tayl le-jiss-LAY-shuhn – The different acts in place are to protect the client, for example the Trades Descriptions Act, the Prices Act, the Sale and Supply of Goods Act, the Consumer Protection Act the Consumer Safety Act and the Data Protection Act.

Consumer Protection Act – kuhn-SYOO-muh pruh-TEK-shuhn akt – A law that protects clients from unsafe products.

Consumer Safety Act – kuhn-SYOO-muh SAYF-tee akt – This act lays down legal safety standards to minimise the risk to the consumer from potentially harmful or dangerous products.

Contact dermatitis – KON-takt dur-muh-TIY-tiss – A skin condition that can be sore, red and itchy.

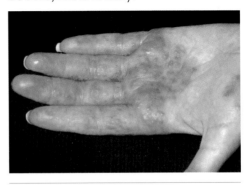

Contagious – kuhn-TIY-juhss – A contra-indication that can be passed on to another person.

Contaminated waste – kuhn-TAM-in-ay-tid WAYST – Consumables that have been soiled with bodily fluids; this type of waste requires special disposal methods.

Contamination – kuhn-ta-mi-NAY-shuhn – The presence of something unwanted that might be harmful.

Contingency plan – kuhn-TIN-juhn-
see PLAN – Back-up or secondary plan.

Continuing professional development (CPD) – kuhn-TIN-yoo-ing pruh-FESH-uh-nuhl duh-VEL-uhp-muhnt -- SEE-PEE-DEE – The term used to describe how people in a profession continue to update and improve their skills throughout their career.

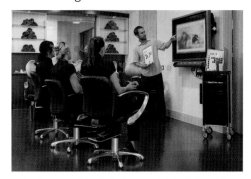

Contra-action – KON-truh-AK-shuhn – An unwanted reaction occurring during or after treatment.

Contra-indication – KON-truh-in-di-KAY-shuhn – The presence of a condition that may prevent or restrict the treatment taking place.

Contract of employment – KON-trakt uhv im-PLOY-muhnt – A legal document, which details such things as salary, holidays and working hours.

Contraction – kuhn-TRAK-shuhn – When the muscle shortens and thickens, and in doing so creates a joint movement.

Contractor – kuhn-TRAK-tuh – A person who isn't directly employed by a business but does have a contract with them to complete work by a set deadline. For example, a builder.

Contractual agreement – kuhn-TRAK-tyoo-uhl uh-GREE-muhnt – This is a verbal or written agreement undertaken by you, the salon and the client to carry out the agreed standard of service, providing the benefits discussed at the agreed price.

Control – kuhn-TROHL – The elimination or reduction of the risk to acceptable levels.

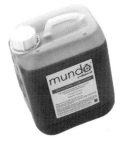

Control of Substances Hazardous to Health (COSHH) – kuhn-TROHL uhv SUB-stuhn-siz HAZ-uh-duhss tuh HELTH -- KOSH – Health and safety regulations require employers to identify hazardous substances used in the workplace and state how they should be stored and handled.

Copolymer – koh-PO-li-muh – A polymer made from two or more different monomers.

Copyright – KO-pee-riyt – The legal right that gives the creator of a piece of work control over how it is used by others.

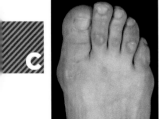

Corn – KORN – Usually found on the toes and feet, this is a small area of thickened skin. It is often caused by pressure or friction to the area, eg shoe rubbing.

Cornea – korn-EE-uh – The clear front window of the eye that transmits and focuses light into the eye.

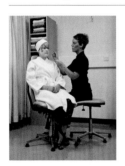

Correct posture – kuh-REKT POSS-chuh – Positioning yourself correctly to prevent fatigue and long-term injury.

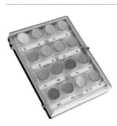

Corrective colours – kuh-REK-tiv KUH-luhz – Make-up products used to balance the skin tone.

Corrugator – KO-ruh-gay-tuh – Facial muscle found between the eyebrows.

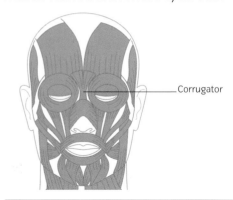

Corrugator

Cortex – KOR-teks – The middle layer of the hair where the pigment melanin is found.

Cosmetic enhancement – koz-MET-ik in-HAHNSS-muhnt – An application technique which improves the appearance of a damaged nail.

Cost-effective – KOST-if-FEKT-iv – Achieving a style at good value for money.

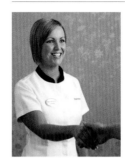

Courteous behaviour – KURT-ee-uhss bi-HAY-vee-uh – Treating your client politely and showing them respect.

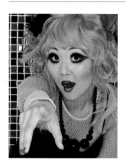

Creative skills – kree-AY-tiv SKILZ – Using your imagination and artistic flair when creating new fashion trends.

Cross-contamination – KROSS-kuhn-ta-mi-NAY-shuhn – When micro-organisms are allowed to come into contact with a surface/substance.

Cross-infection – KROSS-in-FEK-shuhn – The transfer of micro-organisms through poor hygiene practices by direct contact with another person or indirect contact with infected tools and equipment.

Crystalline coloured enamel – KRISS-tuh-lyn KUH-luhd i-NAM-uhl – This gives a slightly pearlised, shimmery or iridescent appearance; you may need to apply additional coats.

Cultural and fashion trends – KUL-chuh-ruhl uhnd FASH-uhn trendz – Looks that either match fashion changes, or support cultural occasions or needs.

Curing – KYOO-uh-ring – The name used to describe the polymerisation process or the hardening of the acrylic, ie a cured nail is an overlay that has hardened.

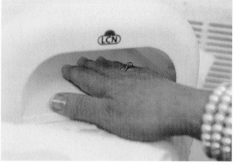

Customer – KUSS-tuh-muh – A person who isn't necessarily a client but has come into the salon to enquire about the services offered or to buy a product.

Cut out – KUT owt – A technique used in advanced nail art. It removes part of a tip to change the original shape.

Cut out method – KUT owt METH-uhd – Where a product is dispensed from a jar/pot using a spatula rather than the fingers.

Cuticle – KYOO-tikl – The overlapping skin at the base of the nail plate, which should be flexible and not overgrown.

Cuticle cream – KYOO-tikl KREEM
– A product used in both manicures
and pedicures to soften and nourish
the cuticles.

Cuticle remover – KYOO-tikl ri-MOO-
vuh – A product used in both manicures
and pedicures to aid the removal of
cuticles.

Cyanoacrylate – siy-an-oh-AK-ri-
layt – A family of chemicals known as
'acrylates' that are used in adhesives
and resins.

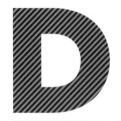

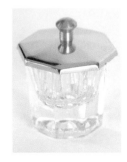

Dappen dish
– DAP-uhn DISH –
A small container
used to hold liquid
products while
working.

Dark circles – DAHK SURKLZ –
Areas of darker skin colour found
under the eyes.

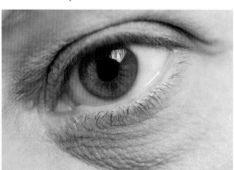

Data Protection Act – DAY-tuh pruh-
TEK-shuhn akt – Legislation designed
to keep clients' personal details private.
You need to know how this affects your
work, and what you must and must not
do to comply with it.

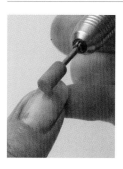

De-bulking
– dee-BUL-king
– Reduction of the nail overlay prior to rebalance.

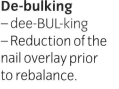

Debit card
– DEB-it KAHD – A means of making payment without cash; the money instantly leaves the client's bank account.

Debris – DEB-ree – This is the excess of a material that is not used, eg excess face mask when carrying out a facial.

Decant – dee-KANT – To pour liquid from one container to another, usually from a larger container to a smaller container.

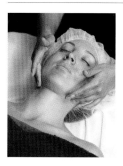

Décolleté
– day-KOL-tay – The area between the neck and bust where the skin is much thinner and almost always exposed to the environment.

Deep vein thrombosis (DVT) – DEEP VAYN throm-BOH-siss -- DEE-VEE-TEE
– A blood clot that develops in a deep vein, causing pain and swelling. It can break away and travel to other areas of the body. The lungs and heart are often affected. DVT can be fatal.

Defects – DEE-fekts – This applies to damaged products and packaging, such as leaking containers or loose packaging.

Dehydrated – dee-hiy-DRAY-tid – A skin condition where the surface lacks moisture and water. The skin will appear tight and parched, often with very fine lines.

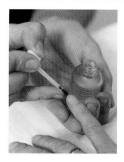

Dehydrator
– dee-hiy-DRAY-tuh – A product used to remove water or dry out the nail plate.

Delamination – dee-lam-i-NAY-shuhn – Where the nail plate layers have separated from each other causing peeling and splitting. This is usually caused by a combination of dryness and trauma to the free edge.

D

Deltoid – DEL-toyd – Muscle that covers the shoulder and assists with lifting the arm and moving it back and forwards.

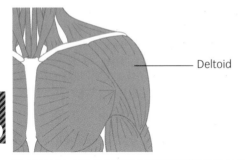

Deltoid

Demonstration – dem-uhn-STRAY-shuhn – A teaching or marketing presentation to increase client understanding and interest in a product or service.

Deodorant – dee-OH-duh-ruhnt – Used to prevent underarm and foot odour.

Depilation – dep-i-LAY-shuhn – Temporary method of removing hair, eg waxing, shaving and depilatory creams.

Depilatory creams – duh-PIL-uh-tree KREEMZ – Chemical creams that dissolve the hair on the surface of the skin.

Depressor labii – duh-PRESS-uh LAY-bee-ee/LAY-bee-iy – Muscle that runs down the chin from the lower lip.

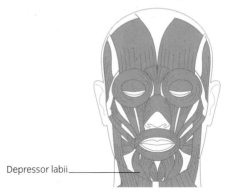

Depressor labii

Dermal cord – DUR-muhl KORD – Where a new hair germ cell begins its life.

Dermal fillers – DUR-muhl FIL-uhz – These add volume to the face and, depending on the type of filler and the depth injected, fine lines can be smoothed and deep lines filled. They can also be used to plump up areas such as the lips.

Dermal papilla – DUR-muhl puh-PILL-uh – The base of the follicle is attached to the blood supply and provides oxygen and nutrients, stimulating hair growth throughout the anagen phase.

Dermatitis – dur-muh-TIY-tiss – A common skin condition suffered by beauty therapists, when wet work and contact with chemicals cause soreness, redness and itchiness to the skin.

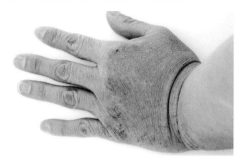

Dermatosis papulosa nigra – dur-muh-TOH-siss pap-yoo-LOH-suh NIY-gruh – Non-infectious and non-cancerous lesions that develop in the pilosebaceous unit of the skin.

Dermis – DUR-miss – The layer under the epidermis, which contains collagen and elastin fibres.

Design objective – di-ZIYN uhb-JEK-tiv – The aim or desired end result of the make-up.

Design plan – di-ZIYN PLAN – This is a written outline of how you plan to achieve the desired effect. You present this to the person who has set you the task for their approval.

Desincrustation – dess-in-kruss-TAY-shuhn – A treatment using a negatively charged galvanic current to break down the acid mantle, soften keratin, dilate pores and saponify sebum to make deep extraction work possible.

Desirable characteristics – di-ZIY-ruhbl karr-ik-tuh-RISS-tiks – The appropriate conditions that are needed to carry out a skin tanning treatment such as warmth, ventilation, privacy and music.

Desquamation – dess-kwuh-MAY-shuhn – The skin's own natural exfoliation process: the shedding of the top layers of the stratum corneum.

Development time – duh-VEL-uhp-muhnt TIYM – A term used in self-tanning to describe how long the product should be left on in order to produce the tan. It will vary between manufacturers, but is usually 4–6 hours. The term is also common in eyelash perming or tinting.

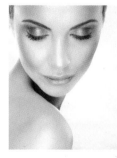

Dewy make-up – DYOO-ee MAYK-up – A popular summer look that provides a shimmer to the skin, enhancing natural features with frosted highlighters and tints. Use cream, liquid and gel products rather than powders. This look is particularly suited for those going on beach holidays and those with blemish-free complexions.

Diabetes – diy-uh-BEE-teez – A medical condition that contra-indicates waxing as the skin can lose sensation, bruise easily and heal poorly.

Diabetes type 1 – diy-uh-BEE-teez TYP WUN – This type of diabetes is insulin dependent as the body makes little or no insulin.

Diabetes type 2 – diy-uh-BEE-teez TYP TOO – This type of diabetes is initially controlled by diet and tablets because the blood sugar levels are unbalanced.

Diagnosis – diy-uhg-NOH-siss – Observing and identifying a disease or disorder.

Diamond bits – diy-uh-muhnd BITS – Made from diamond particles that scratch the surface of the overlay, producing a very fine dust.

Diathermy – DIY-uh-thur-mee – Often referred to as SWD (short wave diathermy). The fastest method of epilation, it uses an alternating oscillating current to produce heat that either coagulates or cauterises the tissues.

Digestive system – diy-JESS-tiv SISS-tuhm – This includes all the structures that are needed to digest food.

Digitorum longus extensor – dij-i-TOR-uhm LONG-giss iks-TEN-suh – Muscle that makes up the outer edge of and just behind the tibialis anterior, extending from the outer edge of the knee to the outside of the ankle.

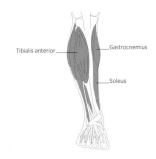

Tibialis anterior — Gastrocnemius — Soleus

Dihydroxyacetone (DHA) – diy-hiy-DROK-see-ASS-uh-tohn -- DEE-AICH-AY – A sugar found in self-tanning products that reacts with amino acids in the skin to produce a tanned effect.

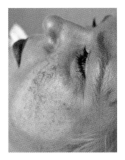

Dilated capillaries – diy-LAY-tid kuh-PILL-uh-riz – Fine red lines that show through the skin; often found on sensitive fine skin on the cheeks or around the nostrils. Sometimes referred to as thread veins.

Direct current – diy-REKT KURR-uhnt – A current that is constant and flows in one direction.

Direct high frequency – diy-REKT HIY FREE-kwuhn-see – A treatment using ozone to control an oily, pustular or acnied skin.

Direction of growth – diy-REK-shuhn uhv GROHTH – The direction the hair grows up through the follicle and out on to the skin's surface.

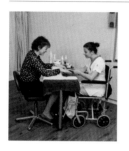

Disability discrimination – dis-uh-BIL-uh-tee dis-krim-i-NAY-shuhn – It is unlawful to discriminate against any person with a disability. For more information, see www.disability.gov.uk.

Disability Discrimination Act – dis-uh-BIL-uh-tee dis-krim-i-NAY-shuhn akt – This protects people and makes it unlawful to discriminate against a person with a disability on the grounds of his or her disability. This is in relation to recruitment, promotion, training, benefits, or terms and conditions of employment and dismissal.

Disciplinary procedure – diss-ip-LIN-uh-ree pruh-SEED-yuh – Employers use disciplinary procedures to tell employees that their performance or conduct isn't up to the expected standard, and to encourage the employee to improve.

Discrepancies – diss-KREP-uhn-sizz – A term used when handling money. The discrepancy might be an invalid credit card, invalid currency, suspected fraudulent payments using a card, etc.

Discussion – diss-KUSH-uhn – A conversation between the client and the therapist to determine the client's needs.

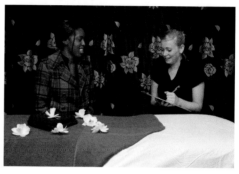

Disinfectant – diss-in-FEK-tuhnt – A substance capable of removing or reducing micro-organisms.

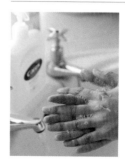

Disinfecting hands – diss-in-FEK-ting HANDZ – Washing the hands to an antiseptic level to limit the presence of bacteria.

Disinfection – diss-in-FEK-shuhn – This limits the growth of disease causing micro-organisms using chemical agents.

Display – diss-PLAY – An arrangement of products and other media to attract attention.

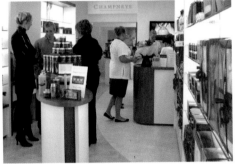

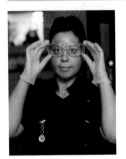

Disposable gloves – diss-POH-zuh-buhl GLUVZ – Part of the PPE that a beauty therapist will wear, often in the form of powder-free, nitrile or vinyl.

Disposables – diss-POH-zuh-buhlz – Single-use products and equipment, such as paper towels, cotton pads, orange wood sticks, unwashable files and buffers.

Disposal of contaminated waste – diss-POH-zuhl uhv kuhn-TAM-in-ay-tid WAYST – It will be necessary to check the correct disposal of the crystals with your local council, as occasional 'pin prick' bleeding may occur.

Disposal of sharps – diss-POH-zuhl uhv SHAHPS – Sharp items such as needles must be disposed of in a sharps box. Special arrangements are made with the local authority for incineration.

Disposal of waste – diss-POH-zuhl uhv WAYST – Everyday waste such as cotton wool and plastic aprons should be disposed of in a lidded bin with a black plastic bin liner inside it.

Distal – DIS-tuhl – The part of the limb or nail that is the furthest away from the centre of the body.

Distorted follicle – dis-TOR-tid FOL-ikl – A hair follicle that has been distorted, making probing difficult. It is often caused by waxing or aggressive shaving techniques.

Disulphide bonds – diy-SUL-fiyd bondz – These are located in the cortex of the hair. During the eyelash perming process they are broken down and reformed into a new shape, leaving the eyelash with a curl.

Diverse – diy-VURSS – Wide-ranging; different; refers to the differences between people, eg personality, beliefs, religion, race, upbringing and social background.

Divulge – diy-VULJ – Make known to others.

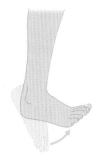

Dorsi flexion
– dor-si-FLEK-shuhn –
Anatomical term where the angle between the toes and the leg decreases when pointing the toes up to the sky.

Double action technique – DUBL AK-shuhn tek-NEEK – Involves depressing the trigger on the top of the airbrush with the index finger to release air only, and drawing it back gradually to the make-up release threshold.

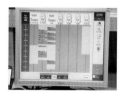

Double booking
– DUBL BUUK-ing – When two clients have been booked in at the same time, owing to an error in the booking system.

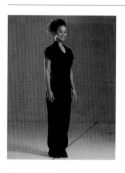

Dress code –
DRESS kohd – The rules around dress/uniform, hairstyle, make-up, nails and jewellery that you are required to follow.

Dry eye syndrome – DRIY IY SIN-drohm – A condition where the eyes don't produce enough tears or they dry out too quickly.

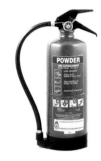

Dry powder extinguisher
– DRIY POW-duh iks-TING-gwish-uh – A red fire extinguisher with a blue band, suitable for burning liquids, such as oil, paint and grease.

Dual action airbrush – DYOO-uhl AK-shuhn AIR-brush – Where the trigger controls both the air and the colour.

Dust extraction – DUST iks-TRAK-shuhn – The mechanical removal of air-borne dust particles in nail treatments.

Dust mask – DUST mahsk – A protective disposable mask worn over the mouth to reduce inhalation of fine dust particles created by using electric files.

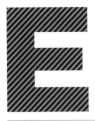

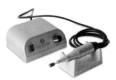

E-file – EE-FIYL – An electric file used on nail overlays to refine, to de-bulk a nail in a maintenance treatment or to buff and create a shine.

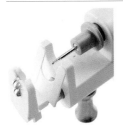

Ear lobe – EER lohb – Contains a lot of blood and keeps the ears warm.

Ear piercing gun – EER PEER-sing GUN – Used to pierce the ear lobes; earrings are placed into the gun, which is spring-loaded.

Eccrine glands – EK-rin or EK-reen or EK-riyn glandz – Sweat glands that are found all over the body, open on the skin's surface and produce sweat.

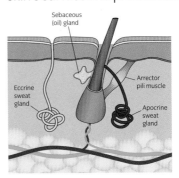

Sebaceous (oil) gland

Arrector pili muscle

Eccrine sweat gland

Apocrine sweat gland

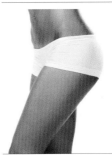

Ectomorph – EK-toh-morf – The body type where the limbs are long and slender, and weight gain is uncommon.

Eczema – EKS-i-muh – Red, irritated, inflamed and itchy skin that is often dry and flaky. Fluid-filled blisters may also appear.

Effective communication – i-FEK-tiv kuh-myoo-ni-KAY-shuhn – Giving and receiving information well, including body language, smiling and tone of voice.

Effective presentation – if-FEK-tiv prez-uhn-TAY-shuhn – When presenting a mood board, you will need to show your planning, include images and colour, show how you have carried out your research, and use your verbal communication and presentation skills.

Effective rapport – if-FEK-tiv ruh-POR – This means getting on well with your clients so they will come back in the future and therefore create more business for your salon.

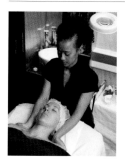

Effleurage – EF-lur-rahzh – A stroking massage technique used to begin the massage, as a link technique, and to complete the facial massage routine.

Eggshell nail – EG-shel NAYL – The nails are thin and fragile with the free edge growing over the tip of the finger.

Elastin fibres – i-LASS-tin FIY-buhz – A protein in the dermis which gives the skin its elasticity and helps to keep it flexible but tight.

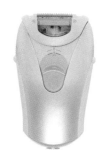

Electrical depilation – i-LEK-trikl dep-i-LAY-shuhn – A temporary form of hair removal using electrical devices, eg 'epilady'.

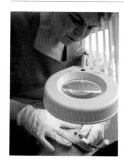

Electrical epilation – i-LEK-trikl ep-i-LAY-shuhn – A permanent method of hair removal, using an alternating high frequency current (referred to as diathermy) to produce heat.

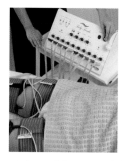

Electrical muscle stimulator (EMS) – i-LEK-trikl MUSSL STIM-yuh-lay-tuh -- EE-EM-ESS – A treatment used to tighten and tone muscles, giving a lifting and slimming effect. Electrical muscle stimulator is used to stimulate motor nerves and muscles. It is sometimes also called body faradic.

Electricity at work regulations
– el-ek-TRISS-it-ee uht WURK reg-yuh-LAY-shuhnz – These regulations state that all electrical appliances must be tested every 12 months by a qualified electrician. It is your responsibility to ensure that you remove any defective electrical equipment, label it as faulty, report it to a responsible person and remove from use.

Electrolysis – uh-lek-TROLL-iss-iss – A permanent method of hair removal, involving chemical destruction of the hair follicle.

Electromagnetic spectrum –
i-LEK-troh-mag-NET-ik SPEK-truhm – Light waves and other types of energy that radiate are called electromagnetic radiation. Together, they form the electromagnetic spectrum. Humans can only see part of the electromagnetic spectrum, for example when a rainbow appears. Energy we can see is called visible light. Ultraviolet light is invisible.

Embedding – im-BED-ing – A nail art technique where three-dimensional designs are created by embedding decorative items.

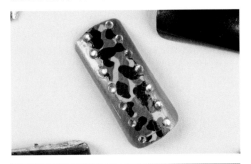

Emergency procedure – i-MUR-juhn-see pruh-SEED-yuh – A plan of movements to evacuate a building. An emergency is a severe, often dangerous situation that needs immediate attention.

Empathy – EM-puh-thee – Understanding how another person feels and reflecting this back to the other person.

Employee – im-ploy-EE – A person who is employed by a business to do work for them.

Employee's basic rights and responsibilities – im-ploy-EEZ BAYSS-ik RIYTS uhnd ruh-sponss-i-BIL-it-eez – The law protects employees from harassment, bullying or any type of discrimination at work. Employers may be taken to court if they do not adhere to the law.

Employer – im-PLOY-uh – A person who owns a business and employs people to work for them.

Employer's liability – im-PLOY-uhz liy-uh-BIL-it-ee – Compulsory insurance that businesses must pay to meet the cost of compensation for any employee injuries or illnesses that occur as a result of their work.

Employer's responsibilities – im-PLOY-uhz ruh-sponss-i-BIL-it-eez – It is the employer's responsibility to provide a safe place of work. They must put into place safety policies and procedures, as well as provide health and safety equipment and training to ensure all employees and anyone entering the salon is kept safe.

Employment Act – im-PLOY-muhnt akt – Covers the right to have statutory leave and pay for maternity/paternity.

Employment Relations Act – im-PLOY-muhnt ruh-LAY-shuhnz akt – Employees have a right to join a trade union. Part-time workers are allowed the same rights as full-time workers.

Employment tribunals – im-PLOY-muhnt try-BYOO-nuhlz – Employment tribunals deal with legal disputes in the workplace. They hear cases involving employment disputes that have not been resolved by other means.

Emulsion – i-MUL-shuhn – A mixture of two or more liquids that don't mix well together naturally. An example is an oil and water.

Endocrine system – END-uh-kreen or END-uh-krin or END-uh-kriyn SISS-tuhm – A system of glands which secrete hormones. These have an effect on particular organs and body systems, and help to regulate the body.

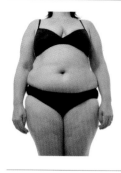

Endomorph – END-oh-morf – The body type where the limbs tend to be short and the hips wider than the shoulders. Weight gain is common.

Energise stones – EN-uh-jiyz STOHNZ – A method used to replace the energies into the stones. This can be done by washing the stones in rain water, leaving them outside overnight (particularly if there is a full moon) or digging and planting the stones into the earth for a period of time.

Enquiries – in-KWIY-uh-riz – Questions that clients may ask to find out about the services offered by a salon.

Environmental conditions – in-viy-ruhn-MENTL kuhn-DISH-uhnz – The work area must be safe and comfortable for employees and clients. Consider heating, lighting and ventilation.

Environmental factors – in-viy-ruhn-MENTL FAK-tuhz – These are the things around you in the salon. An example of a hazard caused by an environmental factor is a wet floor because it may cause someone to slip over on it.

Environmental Protection Act – in-viy-ruhn-MENTL pruh-TEK-shuhn akt – An act for waste management and control of emissions into the environment.

Enzymes – EN-ziymz – Proteins found in fruit that speed up chemical reactions.

Epidermis – ep-i-DUR-miss – The top, outer layer of the skin, which contains five layers. This diagram shows the layers of the epidermis.

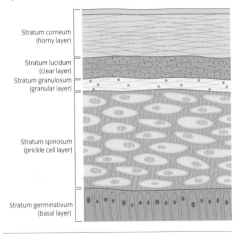

Stratum corneum (horny layer)

Stratum lucidum (clear layer)

Stratum granulosum (granular layer)

Stratum spinosum (prickle cell layer)

Stratum germinativum (basal layer)

Epilepsy – EP-i-lep-see – A neurological condition where there is a tendency for people to have seizures.

Epithelium – e-pee-THEE-lee-uhm – One of the four basic types of tissues that cover the surface of the body.

Eponychium – ep-uh-NIK-ee-uhm – Also known as the cuticle, this is the thickened layer of skin surrounding the fingernails and toenails.

Equal opportunities – EE-kwuhl op-uh-TYOON-it-eez – Nobody should be discriminated against on the grounds of their age, gender or disability. There is legislation to enforce this, and you can see details on this at www.eoc.org.uk.

Equal Pay Act – EE-kwuhl PAY akt – Employers must pay the same rate to men and women for doing the same job of equal value.

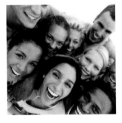

Equality – i-KWOL-it-ee – Treating people the same, regardless of differences like race or gender.

Erector spinae – i-REK-tuh SPIY-nee – A powerful group of three muscles that run down the spine. They help to hold the body upright and extend the spine.

Erythema – err-i-THEE-muh – Reddening of the skin caused by the blood vessels dilating. This may be due to stimulation such as heat or massage, or may occur as an inflammatory response.

Ethical standards – ETH-ikl STAN-duhdz – Working honestly and keeping within all the rules and regulations of your salon and the beauty and nail industry.

Ethmoid – ETH-moyd – One bone between the eye sockets forming part of the nasal cavities.

Ethyl methacrylate (EMA) – EE-thiyl me-THAK-ri-layt -- EE-EM-AY – This monomer is used in nail systems.

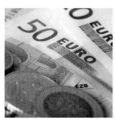

Euro – YOOuh-roh – European currency.

Evacuation procedure – i-vak-yoo-AY-shuhn pruh-SEED-yuh – The exit route and assembly point identified by the salon.

Evaluation – i-val-yoo-AY-shuhn – Measuring how successful or not a promotional activity has been.

Evaluation methods – i-val-yoo-AY-shuhn METH-uhdz – Different ways of getting feedback – these could include team meetings, feedback from your tutor or self-evaluation.

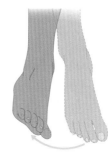

Eversion – i-VUR-shuhn – Anatomical term, meaning to bring the sole outwards.

Evident – EV-id-uhnt – Easily seen.

Excretion – eks-KREE-shuhn – The removal of waste, such as sweat from the skin.

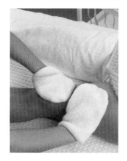

Exfoliation – eks-foh-lee-AY-shuhn – A process to remove dead skin that can be done manually (with hands and product) or mechanically (using a hand-held or electric brush).

Exfoliators – eks-FOH-lee-ay-tuhz – Products used to remove the upper layers of excess skin cells.

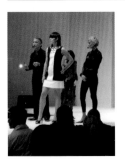

Exhibits – ig-ZIB-its – A way to show or display a fashion or make-up look, company brand, etc.

Exothermic reaction – eks-oh-THUR-mik ree-AK-shuhn – A heat reaction that can occur during polymerisation.

Extension – iks-TEN-shuhn – Anatomical term which means to straighten or bend backwards, making the angle bigger between the joints. An example is straightening the leg at the knee joint.

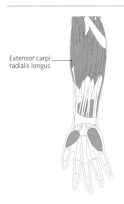

Extensor carpi radialis longus

Extensor carpi radialis longus – iks-TEN-suh KAH-pee/KAH-piy ray-dee-AL-iss LONG-giss – Muscle found in the middle of the forearm. Extends and abducts the wrist.

Extensor carpi ulnaris – iks-TEN-suh KAH-pee/KAH-piy ray-dee-AL-iss ul-NAH-riss – Muscle located to the right of the extensor digitorum muscle. Extends and adducts the wrist.

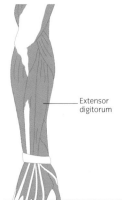

Extensor digitorum

Extensor digitorum – iks-TEN-suh di-ji-TOR-uhm – Muscle that extends from the elbow to the carpals on the back of the forearm. Extends the fingers.

External enquiry – eks-TUR-nuhl in-KWIY-uh-ree – A query that comes from someone outside the salon, for example a phone call from a manufacturer or client.

External obliques – eks-TUR-nuhl oh-BLEEKS – Muscle found on the anterior abdomen. It helps to rotate and laterally flex the abdomen.

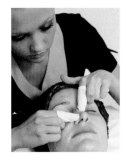

Extraction – iks-TRAK-shuhn – A term used to refer to the removal of comedones or milia using a special tool.

Eye contact – IY KON-takt – Looking someone in the eye when speaking to them (without staring or intimidating them!) is an effective communication tool that will enable you to connect with your colleagues and clients.

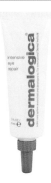

Eye creams/gels – IY KREEMZ/JELZ – Products used around the eye area; ingredients used for specific effects may include moisturising, tightening or line reducing.

Eye products – IY PROD-ukts – Make-up to enhance the eye area, eg eyeshadow, brow colour, eye liner, mascara.

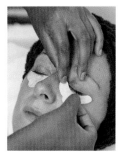

Eye shields – IY SHEELDZ – These can be damp half-moons of cotton wool or pre-prepared pads used to protect the eye area from tint or when applying single lash extensions.

Eye treatments – IY TREET-muhnts – Beauty therapy treatments applied to the eye area to improve the appearance of the eyes.

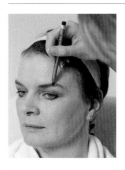

Eyebrow pencil – IY-brow PEN-suhl – Usually comes in either brown, black or grey; it is quite a hard pencil and can give a sharp line.

Eyebrow powder – IY-brow POW-duh – A soft powder applied with a brush or sponge applicator; it comes in a variety of colours, the most popular being black or brown.

Eyelash perming – IY-lash PUR-ming – A treatment used to temporarily curl the upper lashes.

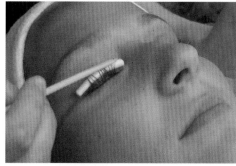

E

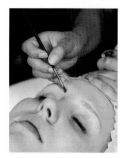

Eyelash/ eyebrow tint – IY-lash/IY-brow TINT – Permanent dye used to colour brow and lash hair. It is made for use around the delicate eye area. It is usually available in blue, black, blue-black, brown and grey.

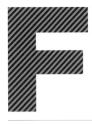

FABs – EF-AY-BEEZ – This stands for Features, Advantages and Benefits, and relates to the links between a product's description, its advantages over others and the benefit the customer will get from using it.

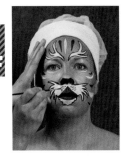

Face painting techniques
– FAYSS PAYN-ting tek-NEEKS – Application of face paints using sponges or brushes.

Face shape – FAYSS shayp – The shape of the client's face. Common ones include square, round, oval, oblong and diamond. This affects the make-up products and techniques that may be used for best results.

Facial – FAY-shuhl – A treatment applied to the skin of the face to cleanse, tone and nourish.

Facial and skull bones – FAY-shuhl uhnd SKUL BOHNZ – The primary bones of the face and skull are the mandible, maxilla, zygomatic, nasal, frontal, parietal and occipital. The point at which bones of the skull are fused together is called a suture.

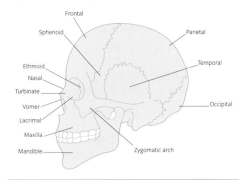

Facial bronzing products – FAY-shuhl BRON-zing PROD-uhkts – Usually in powder form and applied with a brush to give a mild tan effect.

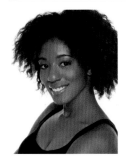

Facial expressions
– FAY-shuhl ik-SPRESH-uhnz – A form of non-verbal communication. Common facial expressions include anger, concentration, confusion, disgust, excitement, empathy, fear, frustration, glare, happiness and sadness.

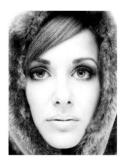

Facial features
– FAY-shuhl FEE-chuhz – Nose, eyes, lips, ears, high/low cheekbones and high/low forehead. These are all taken into consideration when choosing a make-up look for the client; the look will need to complement the client's features.

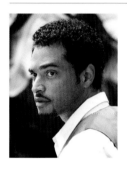

Facial hair
– FAY-shuhl HAIR – The facial hair tends to grow at the lip, cheeks, lower lip, chin and the rest of the lower face to form a full beard.

Facial micro-current – FAY-shuhl MIY-kroh-KUH-ruhnt – A treatment with many benefits including toning, lifting, firming and re-educating muscles, and increasing collagen and elastin production, which slows down skin ageing.

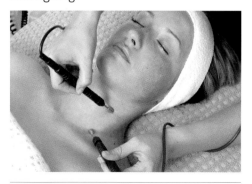

Facial products – FAY-shuhl PROD-uhkts – Preparations applied to the skin to keep it clean, soft, supple and healthy.

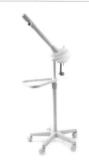

Facial steamer
– FAY-shuhl STEEM-uh – This can be used instead of hot towels in facial massage.

Facial wash – FAY-shuhl WOSH – A cleansing product used with water to cleanse the face, often in gel form.

Facilities – fuh-SIL-it-eez – The facilities in a certain area, eg reception area facilities include the seating area, cloakroom, hot and cold drinks, newspapers and magazines, and retail displays.

False eyelash adhesive – FOLSS IY-lash uhd-HEE-siv – A type of glue used during false lash application to attach the false lashes to the client's natural lashes.

False eyelash solvent – FOLSS IY-lash SOL-vuhnt – A product made to remove single artificial lashes from natural lashes.

False eyelashes – FOLSS IY-lash-iz – Threads of nylon fibres or real hair that are attached to the client's natural lashes. They can be individual, flared or strip.

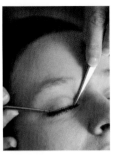

False lash application
– FOLSS lash ap-li-KAY-shuhn – The use of strip or flared lashes that are applied to the client for a special occasion, usually lasting for the evening or, if treated carefully, a week.

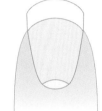

Fan-shaped nail
– FAN-shaypt NAYL – A nail shape where the nail is wider at the free edge.

Faradic current – fuh-RAD-ik KURR-uhnt – A direct, interrupted, surging current used in EMS to cause muscle contraction.

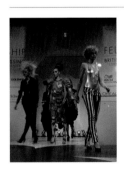

Fashion and photographic settings
– FASH-uhn uhnd foh-tuh-GRAF-ik SET-ingz – Where fashion and photographic events take place, for example fashion shows and magazine shoots.

Fashion stylist – FASH-uhn STIY-list – The person who selects the clothing and accessories for the model. You need to work closely with them, bearing in mind the overall look.

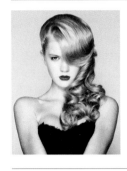

Fashion trends
– FASH-uhn trendz – Current popular styles in clothes, make-up, nail art, etc.

Fatigue – fuh-TEEG – Tiredness or exhaustion.

Features of a product – FEE-chuhz uhv uh PROD-uhkt – Use these to help you sell a product. Eg clients care about the ingredients that the product contains and how it achieves a particular result.

Feedback – FEED-bak – When someone more senior tells you how you are performing at work. This is an essential part of measuring your progress.

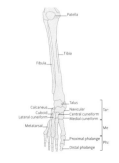

Femur
– FEE-muh – The thigh bone, and the longest bone in the body.

Fibreglass – FIY-buh-glahss – The strong and durable material used in the artificial nail wrap system.

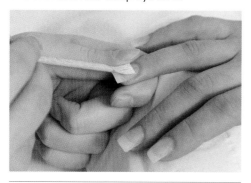

Fibroblasts – FIY-bruh-blasts – Cells found in the dermis that produce new fibrous cells such as collagen and elastin fibres.

Fibromyalgia – fiy-broh-my-AL-juh – A condition that causes musculoskeletal pain. Deep massage on the local area should be avoided.

Fibula – FIB-yuh-luh – A bone located in the lower leg next to the tibia (on the little toe side).

FIFO – FIY-foh – This stands for first in, first out. This refers to a method of stock rotation where older products are used before new products to ensure they do not go out of date.

File attachments – FIYL uh-TACH-muhnts – Found in electric files for nail enhancements, they rotate and come in various shapes, ie barrel bit and cone bit.

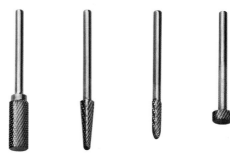

File speed – FIYL SPEED – The speed at which the file rotates, usually between 0–30,000 rpm.

Financial effectiveness of the business – fiy-NAN-shuhl i-FEK-tiv-nuhss uhv dhuh BIZ-niss – The monitoring and effective use of salon resources, and meeting productivity and development targets to make a positive contribution to the effectiveness of the business.

Finnish sauna – FIN-ish SOR-nuh – A dry heat treatment where the air is heated by an electric stove containing coals.

Fire evacuation – FIY-uh i-vak-yoo-AY-shuhn – The instant and speedy movement of people away from the threat of fire.

Fire extinguisher

Fire extinguisher – FIY-uh iks-TING-gwish-uh – There are many different fire extinguishers, classified according to the class of fire for which they should be used. All fire extinguishers are red with a coloured band to show what type of fire it can be used for.

Fire Precautions Act – FIY-uh pri-KOR-shuhnz akt – Employers must train employees in fire safety following a written risk assessment. All equipment and facilities should be regularly maintained and faults rectified as soon as possible. All persons shall be regarded as competent when they have had sufficient training, experience and knowledge to conduct the fire risk assessment.

Fire retardant – FIY-uh ruh-TAH-duhnt – A chemical used to slow down the spread of fire.

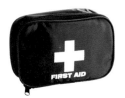

First aid – FURST AYD – Knowing and doing the correct thing if someone has a nosebleed or cut, or in case of an emergency.

First Aid Regulations – FURST AYD reg-yuh-LAY-shuhnz – These regulations require employers to provide adequate and appropriate equipment, facilities and personnel to ensure their employees receive immediate attention if they are injured or taken ill at work. These regulations apply to all workplaces, including those with less than five employees and to the self-employed.

Fitness – FIT-niss – The state or condition of being physically sound and healthy, especially as a result of exercise and good nutrition.

Fitzpatrick classification scale – fits-PAT-rik klass-if-i-KAY-shuhn SKAYL – A method used to classify skin colour and tolerance to sunlight.

Fixing lotion – FIK-sing LOH-shuhn – A chemical, usually sodium bromate, that when applied to the lashes will fix them into their new shape, making the curl permanent.

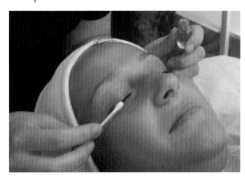

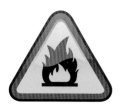

Flammable – FLAM-uh-buhl – Something that will burn quickly when set alight.

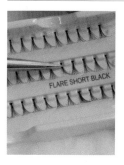

FLARE SHORT BLACK

Flare lashes – FLAIR LASH-iz – A cluster of synthetic lashes applied to the natural lashes. They use a different adhesive from permanent lashes and do not last as long.

Flexion – FLEK-shuhn – Anatomical term which means to bend forwards and make the angle smaller between the joints. An example would be when bending the leg at the knee joint.

Flexor carpi radialis – FLEK-suh KAH-pee/KAH-piy ray-dee-AL-iss – Muscle located above the radius bone. Flexes and abducts the wrist.

Flexor carpi ulnaris – FLEK-suh KAH-pee/KAH-piy ul-NAH-riss – Muscle located above the ulna bone. Flexes and adducts the wrist.

Flexor digitorum – FLEK-suh di-ji-TOR-uhm – Side muscle in the forearm. Flexes the fingers.

Flexor digitorum longus – FLEK-suh di-ji-TOR-uhm LONG-giss – Muscle found on the inside of the back of the lower leg.

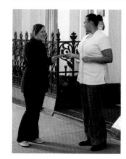

Flier – FLIY-uh – Advertising leaflet often used to promote a service or product.

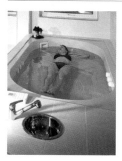

Flotation – floh-TAY-shuhn – A spa treatment where the body is suspended in a bath or tank (wet flotation) or supported on a polymer-covered warmed tank of water (dry flotation), inducing relaxation.

Flow – FLOH – In micro-dermabrasion, the rate at which the crystals flow through the applicator on to the skin.

Fluid retention – FLOO-id ruh-TEN-shuhn – Where the body retains water. It is common around the feet and ankles.

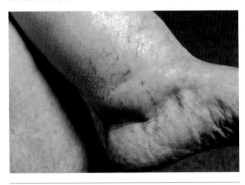

Fluorescent light – fluh-RESS-uhnt LIYT – Intensifies darker tones and softens blues and greys.

Foils – FOYLZ – These are available in many patterns and colours, and can be applied to the nail to give a metallic sheen.

Folliculitis – fo-lik-yoo-LIY-tiss – A bacterial infection of the hair follicle. Appears as a small pustule at the base of the follicle, which is often red and inflamed.

Foot and leg lotion – FUUT uhnd LEG LOH-shuhn – Used to moisturise the skin on the foot and lower leg.

Foot and nail treatments – FUUT uhnd NAYL TREET-muhnts – Specialist treatments that include paraffin wax treatment, foot masks, thermal boots and exfoliators. Several may be used in one treatment.

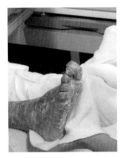

Foot masks – FUUT MAHSKS – Nourishing, moisturising products applied to the feet for a period of time. To increase absorption, feet are placed in hot booties.

Forms – FORMZ – These are applied under the free edge while the nail enhancement is built onto it.

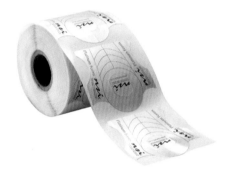

Foundation – fown-DAY-shuhn – Liquid, cream, compact or mousse make-up that contours the face, evens skin tone and disguises minor skin blemishes.

Fraud – FRORD – Deceiving people by using counterfeit money or bank cards. This is a crime.

Fraudulent card – FRORD-yuh-luhnt KAHD – A card that has been stolen or is a fake.

Fraudulent payment – FRORD-yuh-luhnt PAY-muhnt – A debit/credit card, money or a voucher that has been stolen or is a fake.

Free edge – FREE EJ – The white part of the nail that grows beyond the fingertip.

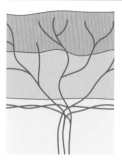

Free nerve endings – FREE NURV END-ingz – Nerve endings that respond to pain and are found just beneath the basement membrane.

Free radicals – FREE RAD-iklz – Substances that attack the cells and tissues, causing damage such as ageing.

Freehand – FREE-hand – Manipulation of the airbrush medium, with air pressure being sprayed without shields or stencils. Can be used for airbrush make-up of nail art designs.

Freelance – FREE-lahnss – Somebody who is self-employed and works independently, for example a make-up artist, mobile therapist or nail technician.

Frictions – FRIK-shuhnz – A type of massage movement where regular pressure is applied to an area, often using static or small circular movements. Frictions help to break down tight muscle fibres.

Frontal – FRUN-tuhl – One bone that forms the forehead.

Frontalis – frun-TAY-liss – This muscle extends over the forehead and raises the eyebrows, wrinkling the forehead.

Full leg wax – FUUL LEG waks – Removing hair from the top of the thighs to the feet (front and back).

Fuller's earth – FUUL-uhz URTH – A natural clay that is used in face masks. It has a deep cleansing and drying effect on the skin.

Functions of the skin – FUNK-shuhnz uhv dhuh SKIN – Shapes: S = sensation; H = heat regulation; A = absorption; P = protection; E = excretion; S = secretion.

Fungus – FUNG-guhss – A fungus is a member of a large group of micro-organisms, many of which will cause diseases.

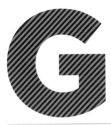

Galvanic burn

Galvanic burn – gal-VAN-ik BURN – Caused by incorrect use of the galvanic machine, this is a chemical burn which looks grey on the skin.

Galvanic current – gal-VAN-ik KURR-uhnt – A constant, direct current where the client forms part of the circuit. It's used in iontophoresis, desincrustation and also in electroylsis hair removal for facial and body treatments.

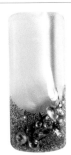

Gamma irradiation – GAM-uh irr-ay-dee-AY-shuhn – A form of sterilisation. It is commonly used for pre-packaged electrical epilation needles.

Gastrocnemius – gass-trok-NEE-mee-uhss – Muscle, more commonly known as the calf muscle.

Gem stones – JEM stohnz – Various little stones that can be adhered to the nail, such as rhinestones, flat stones or pearls.

Gender dysphoria – JEN-duh diss-FOR-ree-uh – A recognised medical condition whereby people view themselves as the opposite sex. Male pattern hair growth is a distressing problem for male-to-female gender dysphoriacs.

General Product Safety Regulations – JEN-ruhl PROD-uhkt SAYF-tee reg-yuh-LAY-shuhnz – This regulation relates to the safe use of all products. Follow all manufacturer's guidance and instructions when using and selling products.

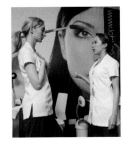

Gestures – JES-chuhz – Hand gestures are commonly used in conversations to emphasise a point.

Glaucoma – glor-KOH-muh or glow-KOH-muh – A group of eye conditions in which the optic nerve is damaged at the point where it leaves the eye.

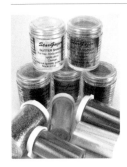

Glitter – GLI-tuh – A heavy, sparkly powder used to give sparkle to the nail.

Gluteals – GLOO-tee-uhlz – Three muscles that form the rear end or bottom. They are the gluteus maximus, gluteus minimus and gluteus medius.

Gluteus maximus – GLOO-tee-uhs MAKS-i-muhss – Muscle that forms the buttocks and extends and rotates the thigh.

Gluteus medius – GLOO-tee-uhs MEE-dee-uhss – Muscle located on the outer surface of the pelvis.

Gluteus minimus – GLOO-tee-uhs MIN-i-muhss – Muscle located below the gluteus medius.

Goodwill and trust – guud-WIL uhnd TRUST – All solid relationships are based on this – it means that there is a mutual liking and understanding between you and the other person. To gain the goodwill and trust of your clients and colleagues, you need to show that you are friendly, helpful and dependable.

Gracilis – GRASS-i-liss – Muscle that runs down the inner leg from the pelvis to the tibia. It adducts the thigh and flexes the leg at the knee.

Gravity feed airbrush – GRAV-it-ee FEED AIR-brush – An airbrush with a small cup attached to the top to hold the paint.

Grievance – GREE-vuhnss – Cause for complaint.

Grievance/Disciplinary procedure – GREE-vuhnss/diss-ip-LIN-uh-ree pruh-SEED-yuh – A set of guidelines to follow in case of complaints, poor performance and misconduct, to ensure fairness to all staff. If you're unsure about your salon's grievance procedures, ask your supervisor.

Grit/abrasive – GRIT/uh-BRAY-siv – In nail enhancements, the higher the grit number, the smoother the file (ie 240 is smoother than 180).

Guidance – GIY-duhnss – To help, seek advice and give direction.

Guide colour – GYD KUH-luh – This is the shade the product looks when first applied to the skin. After development time, it's washed off and the true colour, unique to each client, will be visible.

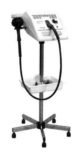

Gyratory massager – JIY-ruh-tu-ree or jiy-RAY-tuh-ree MASS-ah-zhuh or muh-SAH-zhuh – A mechanical massager that has interchangeable heads, each of which gives a different deep massage effect. It can be a free-standing or hand-held appliance.

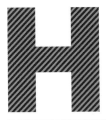

Habia – HAB-ee-ah – The Hair and Beauty Industry Authority; they produce the National Standards that the industry works to.

Habia Code of Practice for Nails – HAB-ee-ah KOHD uhv PRAK-tiss fuh NAYLZ – A set of guidelines by the sector skills body for the nails industry.

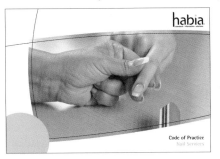

Habia Code of Practice for Waxing – HAB-ee-ah KOHD uhv PRAK-tiss fuh WAKS-ing – A set of guidelines by the sector skills body for the beauty therapy industry.

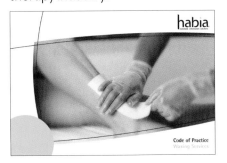

Haemophilia – hee-muh-FIL-ee-uh – A disorder of the blood where there aren't enough platelets to clot the blood where the skin is damaged.

Hair colouring characteristics – HAIR KUH-luh-ring karr-ik-tuh-RISS-tiks – The natural colour of hair. Pigment found in a part of the hair called the cortex gives hair its colour.

Hair follicle – HAIR FOL-ikl – Tube-like depression in the skin which holds the hair and inner root sheath.

Hair growth cycle – HAIR GROHTH SIYKL – The stages of growth, transition and inactivity in the hair follicle.

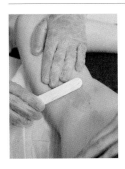

Hair growth direction – HAIR GROHTH duh-REK-shuhn – The direction the hair grows in above the skin's surface.

Hair growth pattern – HAIR GROHTH PAT-uhn – The way the hair grows above the skin's surface. This will be different for each body area but common patterns occur.

Hair shaft – HAIR SHAHFT – The term used to describe the hair above skin level.

Hair tugging – HAIR TUG-ing – A scalp technique where the hair is lifted and pulled at scalp level to stimulate blood flow.

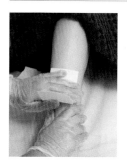

Half leg wax
– HALF LEG waks
– Removing hair from the knees to the front or back of the foot, or from the front/ back of the thighs to the knee.

Halitosis – hal-i-TOH-siss – A term used to describe bad breath.

Hallucis longus extensor – hal-YOO-siss/hal-OO-siss/HAL-uh-kiss LONG-guss iks-TEN-suh – Muscle that runs down the anterior lower leg and extends the big toe.

Hallucis longus flexor – hal-YOO-siss/ hal-OO-siss/HAL-uh-kiss LONG-guss FLEK-suh – Muscle that runs down the posterior lower leg and flexes the big toe.

Hammam – huh-MAHM – A traditional communal type of bath house that is used to detoxify and purify the body, leaving the skin smooth and soft.

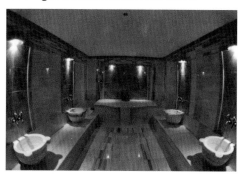

Hammer toes – HAM-uh TOHZ – A deformity of the toes where they start to bend. Often occurs on the second toe.

Hand and nail treatments – HAND uhnd NAYL TREET-muhnts – Specialist treatments that include paraffin wax treatment, hand masks, thermal mitts and exfoliators. Several hand and nail treatments may be used in one treatment.

Hand cream – HAND kreem – Used to moisturise the skin on the hands and lower arms.

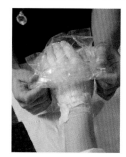

Hand masks – HAND-mahsks – Nourishing, moisturising products applied to the hands for a period of time. To increase absorption, hands are often placed in hot mitts.

Hang nail – HANG nayl – Also referred to as a rag nail. The skin at the nail groove detaches from the nail itself and can become sore.

Hard fat – HAHD FAT – Fat that feels solid to touch. Often found at the tops of thighs.

Hard selling – HAHD SEL-ing – Putting a client under pressure to buy what you're recommending when they don't really want it or feel like they need it.

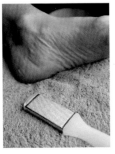

Hard skin – HAHD SKIN – Thick yellowish skin usually found on the sole of the foot where pressure occurs. This is treated after softening the skin, usually with a foot rasp to remove excess dead skin.

Harmonious working relationships – hah-MOH-nee-uhs WUR-king ruh-LAY-shuhn-ships – Working well with your colleagues and understanding the importance of team work. It will help you to work more effectively and create a better impression of your salon to clients.

Hazard – HAZ-uhd – Something that may cause risk of an accident occurring, eg spilt water on the floor.

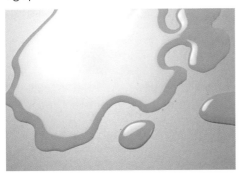

Hazard symbols – HAZ-uhd SIM-buhlz – You might see one or more of these symbols on a single product. They tell us if the product is toxic, corrosive, harmful, explosive, oxidising or flammable.

Hazardous substance – HAZ-uhd-uhs SUB-stuhnss – A product that could harm anyone who comes into contact with it, eg chemicals or cleaning products.

Hazardous waste – HAZ-uhd-uhss WAYST – Waste products such as tissues contaminated with blood. These need to be correctly disposed of to avoid cross-infection.

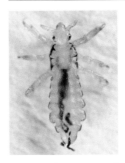

Head lice – HED LIYSS – Also known as pediculosis capitis – head lice are generally spread through direct head-to-head contact with an infested person. The symptoms are itching, red marks and scratch marks on the head. Lice feed on blood from the scalp. The egg or 'nit' may hatch one nymph that will grow and develop to an adult louse.

Health & Safety at Work Act (HASAWA) – HELTH uhnd SAYF-tee uht WURK akt -- AICH AY ESS AY DUBL-yoo AY – This act states the duties of the employer and employee. All the other health and safety laws come under this one.

Health and Safety Executive (HSE) – HELTH uhnd SAYF-tee ig-ZEK-yuh-tiv -- AYCH-ESS-EE – The HSE's job is to prevent people being killed, injured or made ill by work.

Health and safety inspector – HELTH uhnd SAYF-tee in-SPEK-tuh – Health and safety inspectors work to protect people's health and safety, by making sure risks in the workplace are properly controlled.

Health and safety legislation – HELTH uhnd SAYF-tee lej-iss-LAY-shuhn – Laws that outline your responsibilities in protecting the health and safety of your colleagues and clients.

Health and safety policy – HELTH uhnd SAYF-tee POL-iss-ee – The manager of a salon is required by law to draw up a health and safety policy for their business. This must be accessible to all employees, who must read and understand the requirements of the policy.

Heat exhaustion – HEET ig-ZORSS-chuhn – Exhaustion due to the loss of bodily fluids and salts. Symptoms include dizziness, nausea, headaches and fainting.

Heat rash – HEET rash – This occurs when the body is unable to cool itself down. When a person is hot, the body sweats to release excess heat but sometimes this isn't enough and small red pimples form on the skin, usually around the décolleté, neck, elbow crease and groin areas.

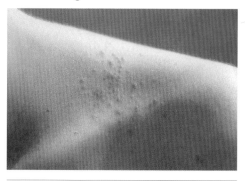

Heat spike – HEET spyk – In nail enhancements, the chemical process of polymerisation is exothermic, ie it releases heat. This problem often occurs during the curing of UV gel. It happens when the polymerisation process occurs too fast under the UV lamp. It's a sudden and painful heat sensation on the nail plate and is alarming for clients. It only lasts a few seconds at the most but it's unpleasant. Modern UV gels have their cure time matched to their recommended UV lamp so it's unlikely to happen. Gels that don't have a dedicated lamp often exhibit this. The way to overcome this is to apply thin layers of gel as thicker layers are more likely to get, a heat spike and less likely to cure fully.

Heat treatments

Heat treatments – HEET TREET-muhnts – Products such as hot oil or paraffin wax, or equipment such as thermal mitts used to heat the hands and aid absorption of products.

Helix – HEE-liks – The prominent rim of the ear. This is made up of cartilage.

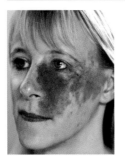

Hemangioma – him-an-jee-OH-muh – A localised, benign skin tumour that is caused by abnormal increase in blood vessels. A common condition is the 'port-wine stain'.

Hereditary – huh-RED-it-ree – Passed on in the genes.

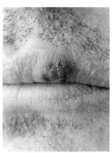

Herpes simplex – HUR-peez SIM-pleks – Commonly known as a cold sore. This is a viral infection where blisters appear around the lip and nose area. They may break open, bleed and crust. In some people, cold sores can be made worse by using a sunbed.

Herpes zoster – HUR-peez ZOS-tuh – Known commonly as shingles, this is a viral infection along the pathway of a nerve. They are common on the face and torso, and can be very painful and cause lesions.

High fashion – HIY FASH-uhn – Make-up which is applied to support the impact of unique, exclusive and trend-setting clothes, often showcased on the runway at international fashion shows.

Highlighter – HIY-liy-tuh – A make-up product that emphasises or draws attention to a certain area.

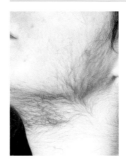

Hirsutism – HUR-syoo-tizm – When a person's hair growth is abnormal for their gender, eg when a female has hair growth on the face that follows the male hair growth pattern.

Histamine (allergic) reaction – HISS-tuh-meen (uh-LUR-jik) ree-AK-shuhn – Histamine is a chemical that is released when the skin comes into contact with a substance to which it is allergic.

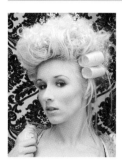

Historical eras
– hiss-TORR-ikl EER-ruhz –
Periods of history such as the 1800s, Egyptian, Roman, Medieval or Edwardian.

Hollywood – HOL-ee-wuud – A term used in female intimate waxing; complete removal of all pubic hair.

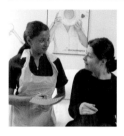

Homecare and aftercare advice
– HOHM-kair uhnd AHF-tuh-KAIR uhd-VIYSS – The advice given to clients to help them keep their style longer; this will include advice on maintenance of the style, tools, equipment and products.

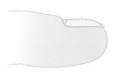

Hooked/claw nail
– HUUKT/ KLOR NAYL – A natural nail plate that curves downwards at the free edge.

Horizontal ridges – horr-i-ZON-tuhl RIJ-iz – Ridges that run from side to side across the nails. Sometimes they are so deep they form furrows.

Hormone – HOR-mohn – A chemical messenger that travels around the body via the blood circulation.

Hospitality – hoss-pit-AL-it-ee – Welcoming the client by offering them refreshments and magazines, and by making sure they are comfortable.

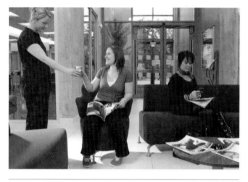

Hot stones – HOT STOHNZ – Stones which are heated in a thermostatically controlled water heater and applied to the body in stone therapies. Basalt stones are commonly used.

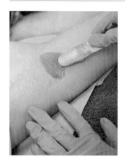

Hot wax – HOT WAKS – A type of wax that is applied in several layers. The first layer is applied against the hair growth using a spatula. After hardening, the end is flicked up and removed against the hair growth.

How to adapt communication –
HOW tuu ah-DAPT kuh-myoo-ni-KAY-shuhn – You need to adapt your communication depending on the situation. Ways to do this are by using different tone and speed, using appropriate terminology, listening and responding appropriately.

Humectant – hyoo-MEK-tuhnt –
A substance, such as glycerol, that attracts moisture. It is added to products to prevent water loss.

Humerus – HYOO-muh-ruhss – The
bone of the upper arm, which is more commonly known as the funny bone.

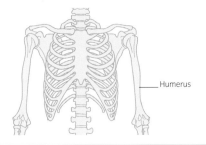

Humerus

Humidity – hyoo-MID-it-ee – This
is the number of tiny water droplets present in the air.

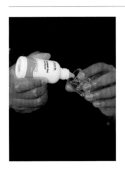

Hydrogen peroxide –
HIY-druh-juhn perr-OK-siyd – A chemical that is mixed with the tint to activate the colour.

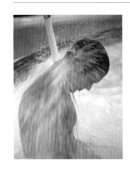

Hydrotherapy
– hiy-droh-THERR-uh-pee – Spa treatments where water is used for its therapeutic effect.

Hygiene – HIY-jeen – Cleanliness.
This is extremely important in a salon, in order to work safely and get the right results.

Hygiene requirements – HIY-jeen
ruh-KWIY-uh-muhnts – The standard expected, as laid down in law, industry codes of practice or written procedures specified by the organisation.

Hygrometer – hiy-GROM-it-uh –
An instrument often used in spas to measure relative humidity.

Hyoid – HIY-oyd – A 'U'-shaped bone
at the base of the neck between the clavicle bones.

Hyper-pigmentation – hiy-puh-pig-men-TAY-shuhn – Increased melanin
production resulting in darker patches of skin compared to other areas.

Hyperaemia – hiy-pih-REE-mee-uh –
The increase of blood flow to different tissues in the body, causing a flushing of the skin.

Hyperkeratosis – hiy-puh-kerr-uh-TOH-siss – Thickening of the skin,
common on elbows and knees.

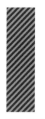

Hypertrichosis – hiy-puh-tri-KOH-siss – When hair growth is considered abnormal for a person's gender, age or race, and may be present at birth (congenital) or appear later in life due to illness, medication or possibly linked to an eating disorder (acquired).

Hypertrophic scar tissue – hiy-puh-TROF-ik SKAH TISH-yoo – This scar tissue is higher than other tissue in the area. It is often referred to as protruding scar tissue.

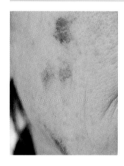

Hypo-pigmentation – hiy-poh-pig-men-TAY-shuhn – The loss of pigmentation in the skin, resulting in paler patches of skin compared to other areas.

Hypodermis – hiy-puh-DUR-miss – A layer of tissue that lies immediately below the dermis of the skin.

Hyponychium – hiy-poh-NIK-ee-uhm – Also known as the quick, this is the soft skin beneath the nail plate that forms a seal to protect the nail bed.

Hypothenar eminence – hiy-POTH-en-uh EM-in-uhnss – This muscle is found in the palm of the hand, lying opposite the thenar eminence. It controls the movement of the little finger.

Ice packs – IYSS PAKS – Cold compresses; may be damp cotton pads or ice wrapped in a small towel. All are used to calm an irritated area.

ICT – IY-SEE-TEE – Stands for information and communication technologies, such as a smart board.

Iliac – ILL-ee-ak – Lymph nodes found in the lower abdomen.

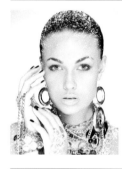

Image – IM-ij – The total look, including hair, make-up, accessories and clothes.

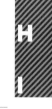

Immune system – i-MYOON SISS-tuhm – The body's defence against infectious micro-organisms, including bacteria, fungi and viruses.

Impetigo – im-puh-TIY-goh – A highly contagious bacterial skin infection normally found amongst pre-school children. It causes painful blisters, usually on the arms and legs.

Implication – im-pli-KAY-shuhn – A likely effect or consequence.

Incandescent light – in-kan-DESS-uhnt liyt – Enhances frosted tones as well as silvers and golds, making it ideal for evening make-up.

Incentives – in-SEN-tivz – Rewards that you get when you've reached your target, which will give you the motivation to work towards them.

Incineration – in-sin-uh-RAY-shuhn – A waste treatment technology that involves the combustion of organic materials.

Incompatible – in-kuhm-PAT-uhbl – Unsuitable.

Indirect high frequency – in-duh-REKT HIY FREE-kwuhn-see – This uses an alternating oscillating current, which flows through both the client and the therapist during facial massage to provide a warming and stimulating effect.

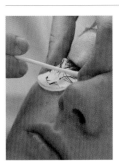

Individual lashes – in-di-VID-yoo-uhl LASH-iz – One or two artificial lashes grouped together to produce a more natural look.

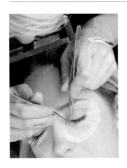

Individual permanent lashes – in-di-VID-yoo-uhl PUR-muh-nuhnt LASH-iz – A process where a single synthetic lash is applied on to a single natural lash using a medical grade long-lasting adhesive. They are used to lengthen the client's natural lashes and can last up to six weeks.

Industry – IN-duh-stree – A type of organised activity that generates money, for example the make-up or nail industry.

Industry sector – IN-duh-stree SEK-tuh – A group of similar industries. For example, hair and beauty is an industry sector.

Infection of the skin – in-FEK-shuhn uhv dhuh SKIN – The growth of micro-organisms caused by bacteria, viruses or fungi. A condition that may cause visible signs of swelling, or redness on the skin, and may spread.

Infectious condition – in-FEK-shuhss kuhn-DISH-uhn – The spreading from one person to another.

Inferior – in-FEER-ree-uh – In anatomy and physiology, this is when something is below or towards the bottom of the body, eg the patella is inferior to the carpals.

Infill – IN-fil – A short nail service, usually performed every two weeks to fill the forward growth at the cuticle area – also known as zone 3.

Inflammation – in-fluh-MAY-shuhn – A condition in which the affected part of the body becomes hot, swollen and sometimes painful.

Influencing factors – IN-floo-uhn-sing FAK-tuhz – Issues, aspects or reasons for designing and carrying out a service in a particular way.

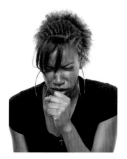

Influenza – in-floo-EN-zuh – Commonly referred to as the flu, the most common symptoms are change in body temperature, coughing, sore throat and headache.

Information required – in-fuh-MAY-shuhn ruh-KWIY-ud – When making an appointment, the receptionist must record the following information: customer's name and contact details, service or treatment required, time of appointment, date of appointment and the name of the person who will provide the service or treatment.

Infrared lamp – IN-fruh-RED LAMP – A lamp that uses infrared light waves, which penetrate the skin, having a warming and relaxing effect. It is usually used on the back before a body massage or to keep the body warm during a body wrap.

Ingrowing toenail – IN-groh-ing TOH-nayl – Also known as onychocryptosis. A common condition where the corners of the nail plate grow into the nail walls, causing swelling and pain.

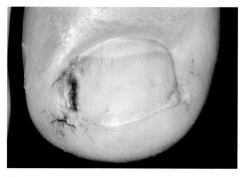

Ingrown hair – IN-grohn HAIR – A hair that grows under the surface of the epidermis and is often curled, forming a spot.

Inguinal – ING-gwin-uhl – Lymph nodes found in the groin region.

Inhibition layer – in-hi-BISH-uhn LAY-uh – In nail enhancements, the surface of the UV gel doesn't cure under the lamp, as oxygen prevents this. When the nails are removed from the lamp, there's a sticky surface. You need to remove this carefully with an alcohol-based cleanser. Uncured gel is a common allergen so take care not to get it on the skin.

Initiator – in-ISH-ee-ay-tuh – The chemical that starts the process of polymerisation.

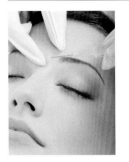

Injectables – in-JEK-tuhblz – Procedures that are administered by syringe and usually into the face, eg Botox.

Instructional techniques – in-STRUK-shuhn-uhl tek-NEEKS – Used to present and instruct information, eg skills demonstrations, diagrams, written instructions, verbal explanations.

Instructions – in-STRUK-shuhnz – A detailed description of how to carry out a service or how to use a product.

Insulated needle – IN-syuh-lay-tid NEEDL – A needle with a coating covering the shaft, leaving only the tip exposed.

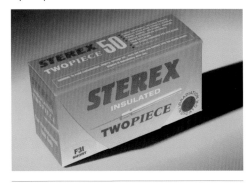

Insurance – in-SHOH-ruhnss – Protection for you and your business; this can include public liability insurance professional indemnity insurance and employer's liability.

Intensive pulse light (laser) – in-TEN-siv PULSS liyt (LAY-zuh) – An electrical piece of equipment used for a variety of treatments including hair removal, reduction of skin blemishes, reduction in scar tissue and improving the overall appearance of the skin. It uses a special lamp that beams light in pulses on to the skin and through the top layers.

Intermediate colour – in-tuh-MEED-ee-uht KUH-luh – One primary colour mixed with one secondary colour equals an intermediate colour.

Internal enquiry – in-TUR-nuhl in-KWIY-uh-ree – A question that comes from someone inside the salon, for example a client enquiring about appointment availability.

Internal obliques – in-TUR-nuhl oh-BLEEKS – Muscle found on the anterior abdomen. It helps to rotate and laterally flex the abdomen.

Internal quality insurance – in-TUR-nuhl KWOL-it-ee in-SHOH-ruhnss – This a system of quality checks made by someone in the centre to ensure that assignments have been written correctly and that assessment decisions are accurate. It is a recorded discussion between two professionals to ensure accuracy, fairness, consistency and quality of assessment. It does not involve the learner.

Interrupted direct current – in-tuhrr-UP-tid diy-REKT KURR-uhnt – A current that flows in one direction but has periods of no current flow. It is used in EMS.

Invalid card – in-VAL-id KAHD – A card that has expired or has been refused due to lack of funds in the client's bank account or because the client has exceeded their credit limit.

Invalid currency – in-VAL-id KURR-uhn-see – Currency from another country, or old versions of coins and notes, that cannot be used.

Inventory – IN-vuhn-tree or in-VENT-uh-ree – A list of the goods you have in stock.

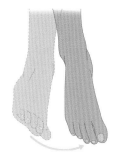

Inversion – in-VUR-shuhn – Anatomical term meaning to bring the sole of the foot inwards.

Involuntary muscles – in-VOL-uhn-tree MUSSLZ – Muscles that contract without any effort from a person, eg the walls of the bladder when we go to the toilet.

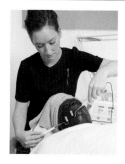

Iontophoresis – iy-on-toh-fuh-REE-siss – A treatment using a direct galvanic current where the selected product is 'pushed' into the skin using a charged electrode.

Irritant – IRR-it-uhnt – A substance, product or chemical that damages the skin and makes it inflamed.

Irritant contact dermatitis – IRR-it-uhnt KON-takt dur-muh-TIY-tiss – This skin condition can develop at any time. The symptoms are dryness, redness, itching, flaking/scaling, cracking/blistering and pain. You can help to prevent contracting dermatitis by wearing non-latex disposable gloves when using any colouring product.

Isometric contraction – iy-suh-MET-rik kuhn-TRAK-shuhn – Equal length; the length of the muscle does not change but there is a change in tone.

Isopropyl alcohol – iy-soh-PROH-pil AL-kuh-hol – Widely used as a cleaning fluid, especially for dissolving oil.

Isotonic contraction – iy-suh-TON-ik kuhn-TRAK-shuhn – Equal tone; the muscle changes in length throughout the movement but the tone remains the same.

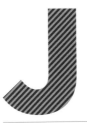

Jade stone – JAYD-stohn – A cold disc onto which the adhesive is dispensed. It keeps the adhesive a constant temperature throughout the treatment.

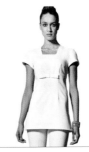

Job description – JOB diss-KRIP-shuhn – An explanation of a person's specific job role, duties and responsibilities.

Job responsibilities – JOB ruh-spon-suh-BIL-it-eez – A detailed list of all the jobs you will be required to undertake.

Job roles – JOB ROHLZ – The tasks and responsibilities that each person in the workplace is there to carry out.

Junior therapist – JOO-nee-uh THERR-uh-pist – A therapist qualified up to Level 2 treatments. It may also refer to a newly qualified therapist when they first start work.

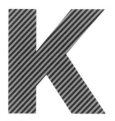

Kabuki brush – kuh-BOO-kee brush – Originating from Kabuki theatre in Japan, these are short and wide domed brushes. They are excellent for defining the cheeks and are considered by many to be the brush of choice for mineral make-up and bronzer application.

Keloid scarring/scar – KEE-loyd SKARR-ing/SKAH – A type of scar tissue in which the scar rises above the rest of the skin in a thickened, tomb-like overgrowth of tissue. It is due to the overproduction of collagen.

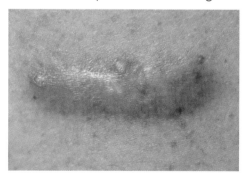

Keratin – KERR-uh-tin – A protein that is a major component of skin, nails and hair. It's present in the epidermis, and there's a high proportion of it in nails and hair where the cells have become keratinised.

Keratinisation – kerr-uh-tin-iy-ZAY-shuhn – The hardening of a cell caused by the production of a protein called keratin and the degeneration of its nucleus.

Koilonychia – koy-loh-NIK-ee-uh – More commonly known as a spoon-shaped nail. This is where the nail curves upwards like a spoon.

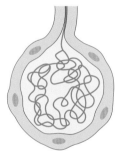

Krause corpuscles – KROW-zuh KOR-pusslz – Nerve endings that respond to cold and are found midway in the papillary region.

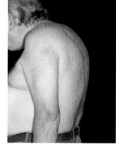

Kyphosis – kiy-FOH-siss – A postural condition where the upper thoracic area of the spine curves forward, rounding the shoulders and causing the head to 'poke' forward.

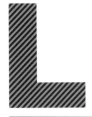

L-Tyrosine – EL-TIY-ruh-seen – A tan accelerator that helps with the skin's own production of melanin.

Laconium sauna – luh-KOH-nee-uhm SOR-nuh or SOW-nuh – A type of sauna that uses underfloor heating to create a mild form of dry heat. It is often more tolerable than the Finnish sauna.

Lacrimal – LAK-rim-uhl – Two bones that form the inner wall of the eye socket.

Lactic acid – LAK-tik ASS-id – A waste product produced by the muscles during stress, exercise and fatigue.

Lanugo hair – luh-NYOO-goh HAIR – Fine, downy hair that is often found on a newborn baby.

Las Vegas – LASS VAY-guhss – A Brazilian, Playboy or Hollywood wax effect decorated with diamanté.

Lash adhesive – LASH uhd-HEE-siv – A glue that is used to ensure the artificial lashes 'stick' and remain in place.

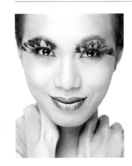

Lash extension – LASH iks-TEN-shuhn – Advanced technique used to lengthen the client's eyelashes. An individual false lash is attached to an existing lash and will last for up to six weeks.

Lash perming – LASH PUR-ming – Only available professionally, this treatment adds curl and uplift to the lashes.

Lash tinting – LASH TIN-ting – A treatment where the eyelashes are coloured to give them emphasis.

Lateral – LAT-uh-ruhl – An anatomical term meaning towards the outer side of the body, eg the lateral aspect of the leg is the outer side of the leg.

Latex – LAY-teks – A common ingredient in peeling masks, making them pliable so they don't crack.

Latex glove – LAY-teks GLUV – You should avoid using this kind of glove, as many people are allergic to latex.

Latissimus dorsi – la-TISS-i-muhss DOR-see – A large muscle that covers the back; it adducts and rotates the arms.

Layers – LAY-uhz – The three layers of the hair are like a pencil. The cuticle is like the varnish on the outside of a pencil, which sometimes gets a little flaky. The cortex is like the wood in the pencil, giving it strength, and the medulla is like the lead.

Legal requirements – LEE-guhl ruh-KWY-uh-muhnts – Working practices and conditions specified by local or national law.

Legal tender – LEE-guhl TEN-duh – Money that is legal in a given country.

Legionnaires' disease – lee-juhn-AIRZ diz-EEZ – A type of pneumonia caused by the inhalation of water droplets contaminated with the Legionnella pneumophila bacterium. This is a potentially fatal disease but is easy to prevent by maintaining high standards of hygiene in wet areas. Legionnaires' disease can be found in wet areas with stagnant water. Air conditioners and humidifiers also carry the risk of this disease. For more information, read the HSE information handbook.

Legislation – lej-iss-LAY-shuhn – Laws affecting the business and its operation, treatments, the working environment, employees and systems of work.

Lentigines – len-TIJ-in-eez – Often referred to as liver spots or age spots, these are large pigmented freckles commonly found on the back of the hands, face and upper back.

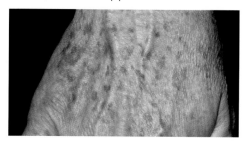

Lethargy – LETH-uh-jee – A feeling of tiredness and indifference.

Leukonychia – loo-kuh-NIK-ee-uh – Commonly mistaken to be a calcium deficiency when it's simply a trauma to the nail. It causes air bubbles between the keratin layers and is identified as white spots on the nail plate.

Levator labatis – luh-VAY-tuh luh-BAY-tiss – Muscle that forms the sides of the upper lip.

Levator scapula – luh-VAY-tuh SKAP-yuu-luh – Muscle found at the back and sides of the neck. It helps to lift the shoulder.

Lifestyle – LIYF-stiyl – Any aspects of a client's life, such as job, hobbies and family situation, that need to be considered when completing a consultation with a client.

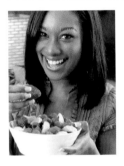

Lifestyle patterns – LIYF-stiyl PAT-uhnz – Habits including smoking, alcohol intake, sleeping, relaxation and exercise patterns, and diet and fluid intake.

Lifting – LIF-ting – When the overlay lifts from the nail plate. It can be seen as a whitish area usually at the base of the nail in the cuticle area. It weakens the nail enhancement but, more importantly, allows bacteria to enter the space under the overlay. This is an ideal environment for bacteria to grow as it's warm and moist. After a few days, a yellow stain will appear. This, if left unchecked, will darken to almost black. This is sometimes known as pseudomonas.

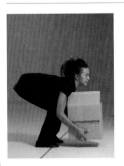

Lifting objects – LIFT-ing OB-jekts – When lifting heavy objects, you have to consider the health and safety risk. The Manual Handling Regulations are designed to protect you and minimise risks relating to the lifting and handling of heavy goods.

Limbic system – LIM-bik SISS-tuhm – The area of the brain concerned with instinct, memory and behaviour.

Limescale – LIYM-skayl – This is a hard, off-white, chalky deposit. It is often found in the bottom of kettles.

Limited company – LIM-it-id KUM-puh-nee – A company that has shareholders.

Limits of authority – LIM-its uhv orth-ORR-it-ee – This describes work that you are not allowed to do in your salon, such as dealing with refunds on reception. You must refer these to a senior team member.

Line manager – LIYN MAN-i-juh – Someone who heads a department and is responsible for achieving the department's objectives.

Link-selling – LINK-SEL-ing – The recommendation of products and services to meet a client's needs and enhance their experience.

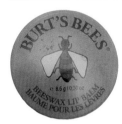

Lip creams/balms – LIP-kreemz/LIP-bahmz – Products used around the lip area; ingredients used for specific effects may include lip plumping, line reducing or nourishing.

Lip products – LIP PROD-uhkts – Make-up that defines, enhances and colours lips, eg lip liner, lipstick, lip gloss.

Liquid and powder – LIK-wid uhnd POW-duh – Used in nail enhancements. Often referred to as acrylic but its correct term is liquid and powder. This system is a two-component system that uses monomer (liquid) and a polymer (powder) mixed together to create a chemical reaction (polymerisation) that produces a solid nail structure.

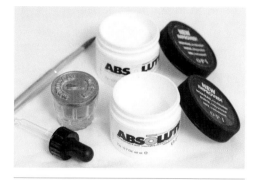

Liquid latex – LIK-wid LAY-teks – Used to create artificial skin and scarring effects. When wet, the solution is in liquid form but it dries to a solid, flexible form.

Local by-law – LOH-kuhl BY-LOH – A local council rule.

Local Government (Miscellaneous Provisions) Act 1982 – LOH-kuhl GUV-uhn-muhnt (miss-uh-LAY-nee-uhss pruh-VIZH-uhnz akt) NIYN-teen AY-tee-TOO – This requires salons performing cosmetic skin piercing such as ear piercing to register with their local authority.

Longevity of tan – lon-JEV-uh-tee uhv TAN – The length of time that the tan lasts before fading.

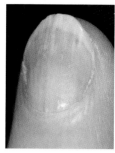

Longitudinal ridges – long-gi-TYOO-din-uhl or lon-ji-TYOO-din-uhl RIJ-iz – Ridges that run from the cuticle to the free edge of the nail; very common on the toenails.

Longitudinally – long-gi-TYOO-din-uhl-lee or lon-ji-TYOO-din-uhl-lee – Along the length of a nail, from the cuticle to the free edge.

Lordosis – lor-DOH-siss – A postural condition where the lower lumbar region of the spine curves in, causing a 'hollow' back and the buttocks and abdomen to protrude.

Lower arch – LOW-uh AHCH – The curve of the lower underside of the free edge when checking the nail from the side profile.

Lubricant – LOO-brik-uhnt – A product that contains oils, making the external surface of the skin feel greasy and slippery.

Lunula – LOON-yuh-luh – The crescent-shaped whitish area of the bed of the fingernail or toenail.

Lymph – LIMF – A yellow-coloured fluid that derives from blood plasma. It transports waste and some fat particles, flowing in one direction from the tissue cells, and to the right and left into the subclavian veins.

Lymph nodes – LIMF nohdz – These are made up of lymph tissue; they are found around the body and filter lymph.

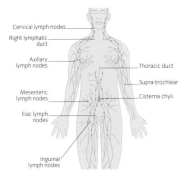

Cervical lymph nodes
Right lymphatic duct
Axillary lymph nodes
Mesenteric lymph nodes
Iliac lymph nodes
Thoracic duct
Supra-trochlear
Cisterna chyli
Inguinal lymph nodes

Lymph vessels – LIMF VESS-uhlz – These carry lymph from the capillaries to the subclavian veins.

Lymphatic drainage equipment – lim-FAT-ik DRAY-nij i-KWIP-muhnt – Equipment developed to increase and stimulate the lymphatic flow. A common piece of equipment is the vacuum suction machine.

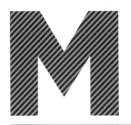

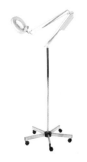

Magnifying lamp – MAG-ni-fiy-ing LAMP – A lens that magnifies the area and also has a light that allows the therapist to see more clearly.

Maintenance – MAYN-tuh-nuhnss – The term used when the client returns to the salon every two to three weeks and has the nails reshaped, rebalanced, infilled, possibly repaired and the tip repositioned, if appropriate.

Maintenance of tools and equipment – MAYN-tuh-nuhnss uhv TOOLZ uhnd i-KWIP-muhnt– The repair and overhaul of tools and equipment. It also includes performing routine checks to keep the equipment in safe working order and fully functional.

Maintenance treatment – MAYN-tuh-nuhnss TREET-muhnt – A tidy up of the existing brow shape. It might also be a maintenance treatment for nail extensions, which can be a rebalance or a refill.

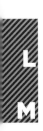

Make-up – MAYK-up – Cosmetics applied to the skin of the face to enhance or disguise the facial features.

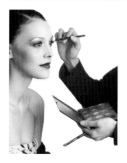

Make-up artist – MAYK-up AH-tist – Someone who uses make-up and specialised techniques to alter or enhance the appearance of others.

Make-up occasions – MAYK-up uh-KAY-zhuhnz – Make-up applied to suit certain events, eg days, evenings or weddings.

Make-up primer – MAYK-up PRIY-muh – A product that is applied instead of moisturiser, when it's unavailable, to provide a velvety texture to the skin so make-up application is smooth and even.

Make-up products – MAYK-up PROD-uhkts – Cosmetics applied to the face to add colour, definition and enhance the client's overall appearance. They should be selected to complement the client's age, skin colour and facial features.

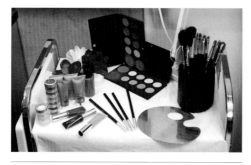

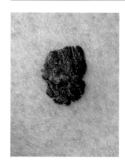

Malignant melanoma – muh-LIG-nuhnt mel-uh-NOH-muh – A form of skin cancer which develops from a mole.

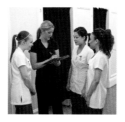

Management – MAN-ij-muhnt – The act of getting people together to achieve desired goals using available resources efficiently and effectively.

Mandible – MAN-dib-uhl – The lower jaw or jawbone.

Manicure – MAN-i-kyoo-uh – Treatments applied to improve the appearance of the hands.

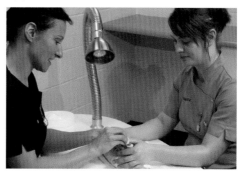

Manicure tools – MAN-i-kyoo-uh TOOLZ – A variety of tools used during a manicure to reduce nail length, carry out cuticle work and shine the nail plate.

Manipulate – muh-NIP-yuh-layt – Handle skilfully, for example manipulating the muscles in a massage.

Mantle – MAN-tl – The deep fold of skin in which the nail is embedded.

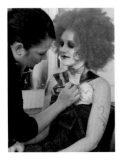

Manual body art techniques – MAN-yoo-uhl BOD-ee AHT tek-NEEKS – Methods of applying body art by hand using sponges and brushes.

Manual Handling Operations Regulations – MAN-yoo-uhl HAND-ling op-uh-RAY-shuhnz reg-yuh-LAY-shuhnz – These regulations are designed to protect you by minimising risks relating to the lifting and handling of heavy goods.

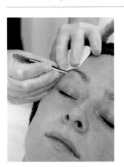

Manual tweezers – MAN-yoo-uhl TWEE-zuhz – Normal tweezers used to remove individual hairs and define the overall shape.

Manufacturer's instructions – man-yuh FAK-chuh-ruhz in-STRUK-shuhnz – Explicit guidance by manufacturers or suppliers on the storage, handling, use and disposal of products, tools and equipment.

Marble – MAHBL – A hard, cold and smooth stone used in stone therapy. Marble is used chilled for its cooling, decongesting and cleansing action, and because it is refreshing and invigorating for the body.

Marbling – MAH-bling – This technique used in nail art involves swirling two or more colours together and can be done with paints, coloured gel or liquid and powder.

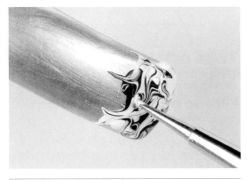

Market research – MAH-kit ruh-SURCH – The collection and analysis of data about a particular target market and competitors in that market.

Marma points – MAH-muh poynts – Pressure points on the body that stimulate life force, similar to acupressure. During Indian head massage you may cover 37 points in the treatment area.

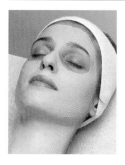

Mask – MAHSK – A skin cleansing product which will contain different ingredients; it can be stimulating, moisturising and toning, and may be either classed as a setting mask, or a non-setting mask.

Massage medium – MASS-ahzh MEE-dee-uhm or muh-SAHzh MEE-dee-uhm – A skin product that moisturises the skin and enables slip and gliding movements to be carried out during a massage routine.

Massage techniques – MASS-ahzh tek-NEEKS or muh-SAHzh tek-NEEKS – These are specific movements applied to achieve a stimulating or relaxing effect, and include effleurage, petrissage, tapotement/percussion, vibration and friction. The speed and depth at which they are applied can alter their effect.

Masseter – mass-EE-tuh – Muscle that runs from the temples to the jaw and works with the temporalis to close the mouth during chewing.

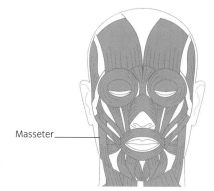

Masseter

Masseur – mass-UR – The term for a male who is qualified in massage.

Masseuse – mass-OEZ – The term for a female who is qualified in massage.

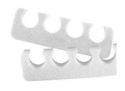

Materials, tools and equipment – muh-TEER-ee-uhlz TOOLZ uhnd i-KWIP-muhnt – Materials include products such as moisturiser and nail polish. Tools include hand-held kit such as tweezers and toe dividers. Equipment includes electrical equipment such as steamers and magnifying lamps.

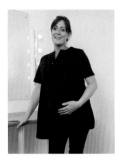

Maternity leave – muh-TUR-nit-ee LEEV – As an employee, you have the right to 26 weeks of Ordinary Maternity Leave and 26 weeks of Additional Maternity Leave, making one year in total. The combined 52 weeks is known as Statutory Maternity Leave.

Matrix – MAY-triks – Where cell mitosis occurs cells divide to make new cells for various structures, eg in the hair, nails and skin.

Mature skin – muh-TYY-uh SKIN – In beauty therapy terms, this is any skin over the age of 25. However, the skin is generally not classed as being mature until the signs of ageing are apparent.

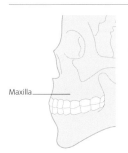

Maxillae – MAK-sil-iy/MAK-sil-ee – Two bones that form the upper jaw.

Maxilla

Media – MEE-dee-uh – The make-up, ornamentations, accessories, video, photographs and clothes that you use.

Medial – MEE-dee-uhl – An anatomical term that means towards the midline of the body, eg the medial aspect of the leg is the inner side of the leg.

Mediate – MEE-dee-ayt – Trying to help resolve an issue between two people or groups.

Medical referral – MED-ikl ruh-FURR-uhl – Referring a particular hair, skin or scalp condition to a specialist to investigate the problem. The referrals should be made to a general practitioner, dermatologist, pharmacist or a trichologist.

Medication – me-di-KAY-shuhn – Treatment with drugs.

Medium – MEE-dee-uhm – A substance that is placed on the body and allows a massage to be carried out, providing slip and glide. These may include oils, creams, emulsions, gels and powders.

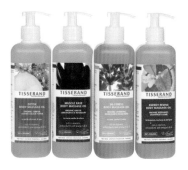

Medulla – me-DUH-luh – The innermost layer of the hair. The medulla gives the hair its sheen as the light is reflected through this layer.

Meibomian gland – miy-BOH-mee-uhn gland – Specialised sebaceous glands at the rim of the eyelids. They secrete sebum to prevent evaporation of the eye's tear film, prevent tear spillage onto the cheek and make the closed lids airtight.

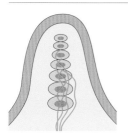

Meissner's corpuscles – MIYSS-nuhz KOR-pusslz – Nerve endings that respond to touch and are found high up in the papillary region.

Melanin – MEL-uh-nin – The dark pigment produced naturally by the skin. Melanin levels vary from client to client, so you'll come across a huge range of skin tones.

Melanocytes – MEL-uh-noh-siyts – Cells that produce melanin, the skin's own natural pigment.

Menopause – MEN-uh-porz – The end of the menstrual cycle. This occurs in women when the ovaries stop producing hormones. The age of menopause varies, but it usually occurs in a woman's late 40s or early 50s.

Menstrual cycle – MEN-stroo-uhl SIYKL – The production of an egg in a woman. If an egg is released but not fertilised the result is blood loss in the form of menstruation.

Mentalis – men-TAY-liss – Muscle under the lower lip in the centre of the chin.

Merkin – MUR-kin – A wig for the pubic region.

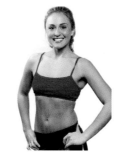

Mesomorph – MES-oh-morf or MEZ-oh-morf or MEE-soh-morf or MEE-zoh-morf – The body type where the shoulders tend to be wider than the hips, and muscle tone is usually well developed.

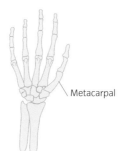

Metacarpals – ME-tuh-KAH-puhlz – Five bones that form the length of the hand.

Metacarpal

Metatarsals – ME-tuh-TAH-suhlz – Five bones that form the length of the foot.

Methods of communication – METH-uhdz uhv kuh-myoo-ni-KAY-shuhn – Your communication with clients may be face-to-face, by letter, fax, phone, email, internet, intranet or any other method you would be expected to use within your job role.

Methods of payment – METH-uhdz uhv PAY-muhnt – The different ways payments can be made, for example cash and debit card.

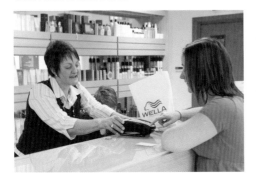

Methods of sterilisation – METH-uhdz uhv sterr-i-liy-ZAY-shuhn – These are the different ways in which high temperature is used to kill off all germs, for example using steam.

Mica – MIY-kuh – Describes the natural colour used in mineral eyeshadows.

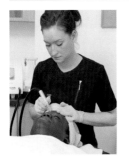

Micro-dermabrasion – MIY-kroh-dur-muh-BRAY-zhuhn – A mechanical exfoliating or skin peeling facial. A controlled, high-speed flow of crystals is applied over the skin's surface.

Micro-lance – MIY-kroh-lahnss – A tiny, sharp, sterile needle used to pierce the epidermis superficially, allowing trapped milia to be removed.

Micro-organisms – miy-kroh-OR-guhn-iz-uhmz – Tiny living beings; they include bacteria, fungi and viruses.

Micro-pigmentation – MIY-kroh-pig-men-TAY-shuhn – A highly skilled treatment where pigment is inserted below the epidermis for cosmetic and/or corrective enhancement.

Milia – MIL-ee-uh – More commonly known as whiteheads, milia are caused by small deposits of fat in the pores that harden and become trapped.

Minimum wage – MIN-i-muhm WAYJ – The minimum amount of money that may be earned per hour, which is set by the Government.

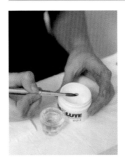

Mix ratio – MIKS RAY-shee-oh – The ratio of liquid to powder in the bead. Used for nail enhancements.

Modification – mod-if-i-KAY-shuhn – Any way you have adapted the treatment to suit client requirements. Always record modifications on the client's record card.

Moisture gradient – MOYSS-chuh GRAY-dee-uhnt – The levels of moisture in the skin (needed for successful epilation) are higher in the deeper levels of the dermis, becoming drier towards the surface.

Moisture trap – MOYSS-chuh TRAP – The glass container that captures any moisture in-between the compressor and the airbrush.

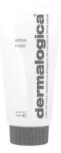

Moisturiser – MOYSS-chu-riy-zuh – A skin care preparation that helps retain natural moisture and adds moisture.

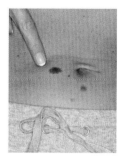

Moles – MOHLZ – Moles are usually a brownish colour, although some may be darker or skin-coloured. They can be flat or raised, smooth or rough; some have hairs growing from them.

Monomer – MON-uh-muh – A liquid used in some nail enhancements. The liquid must mix with the powder polymer to form a solid known as acrylic.

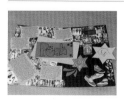

Mood board – MOOD bord – An 'ideas' board showing how a theme is developed.

Motor points – MOH-tuh poynts – Where the motor nerve enters the muscle.

Muscle fatigue – MUSSL fuh-TEEG – A muscle becomes tired and loses the ability to contract efficiently if it runs out of oxygen and glucose.

Muscle insertion – MUSSL in-SUR-shuhn – The moveable, end part of the muscle that moves during contraction.

Muscle origin – MUSSL ORR-i-jin – The fixed position that the muscle starts from. It doesn't move during contraction.

Muscle tone – MUSSL TOHN – The state of partial contraction of a muscle.

Muscles of the face, head and neck – MUSSLZ uhv dhuh FAYSS, HED uhnd NEK – The muscles are frontalis, procerus, nasalis, masseter, zygomaticus, platysma, mentalis, sternocleidomastoid, triangularis, risorius, buccinators, orbicularis oris, quadratus labii superioris, orbicularis oculi, temporalis and corrugator.

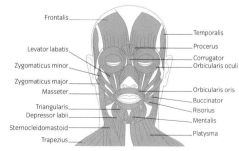

Musculoskeletal disorders – MUSK-yuh-loh-SKEL-itl diss-OR-duhz   Muscle and bone disorders.

Mustard oil – MUSS-tuhd OYL – A popular oil in India and used in Indian head massage. It is very useful during cold spells due to the hot warming sensation it creates. It is good for tense, tight muscles and dryness of the scalp. Not for use on sensitive skin.

Myoblasts – MIY-oh-blasts – When myoblasts fuse together, they form myotubes that eventually develop into skeletal muscle fibres.

Myofibrils – miy-oh-FIY-brilz – Bundles found in the muscles; they are made up of long proteins such as actin and mysoin.

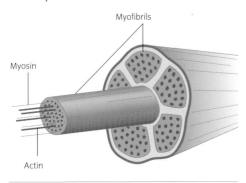

Myofibrils

Myosin

Actin

Myosin – MIY-uh-sin – The commonest protein in muscle cells, responsible for the muscle's elasticity.

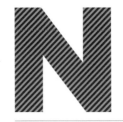

Nail analysis – NAYL uh-NAL-uh-siss – The process of closely looking at the client's nails after wiping over with an antibacterial solution. This is an important activity as the findings are used to create a suitable treatment plan.

Nail and skin products – NAYL uhnd SKIN PROD-uhkts – Used during a manicure or pedicure; they include nail and skin cleanser, nail polish remover, cuticle cream/oil, cuticle remover, buffing paste, hand or foot cream/lotion or oil, base coat, top coat, coloured nail polishes and nail polish drier.

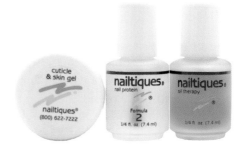

Nail and skin treatment tools –
NAYL uhnd SKIN TREET-muhnt TOOLZ
– Used during a manicure or pedicure;
they include nail files, orange wood
sticks, hoof sticks or cuticle pusher,
cuticle knife, cuticle nippers, foot rasp,
nail buffer and nail scissors.

Nail art – NAYL AHT – Decoration
applied to the natural or artificial nail,
eg nail polish, transfers, gem stones
and glitter.

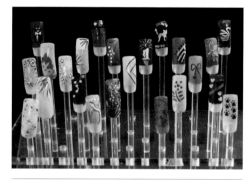

Nail bed – NAYL BED – This can be
found under the nail plate and is made
up of the dermis.

Nail enhancements – NAYL in-
HAHNSS-muhnts – Nail products
applied to the natural nail to artificially
improve its appearance, strength
or length.

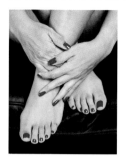

Nail finish –
NAYL FIN-ish –
The finished
result following
a manicure or nail
enhancement
treatment. It will
either be buffed,
French polish
or coloured
nail polish.

Nail groove – NAYL-GROOV – Found
at either side of the nail plate. It holds
the nail plate in place and makes sure it
grows in a parallel line.

Nail growth rate – NAYL GROHTH
RAYT – The rate at which the natural
nail grows.

Nail plate – NAYL PLAYT – The part
of the nail that covers the nail bed –
usually pink in colour.

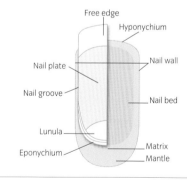

Free edge
Hyponychium
Nail plate
Nail wall
Nail groove
Nail bed
Lunula
Matrix
Eponychium
Mantle

Nail primer – NAYL PRIY-muh –
In nail enhancements, some liquid
and powder and UV gel systems use
a primer. This is a product that prepares
the surface of the nail to create a better
bond with the overlay. Some of them
use methacrylic acid so take care when
you're using this as it's an irritant.
Apply sparingly and always follow the
manufacturer's instructions. Many
modern and good quality systems
don't need a primer, and some UV gel
systems have a specially formulated
base layer instead of a primer.

Nail separation – NAYL se-puh-RAY-
shuhn – When the nail lifts away from
the nail bed.

Nail shapes – NAYL SHAYPS – The shape
that the nail can be filed into, including
oval, square, pointed and round.

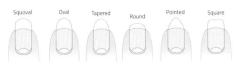

Squoval Oval Tapered Round Pointed Square

Nail structure – NAYL STRUK-chuh –
This is what makes up the nail and
surrounding area.

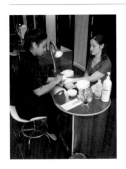

Nail technician
– NAYL tek-NISH-
uhn – A person
who can carry out
a variety of nail
services, for
example
manicures or nail
enhancements.

Nail wall – NAYL WORL – The fold of
skin found at either side of the nail. It
protects the nail plate and the nail bed.

Nail wraps – NAYL RAPS – Fabrics such
as fibreglass and silk with an application
resin are used to overlay the natural
nail. This is often referred to as the
three- or several-component system.

Nasal – NAY-zuhl – Two bones that form
the bridge of the nose.

Nasalis – nay-ZAY-luhss – A muscle
found at the side of the nose. It opens
and closes the nostrils.

National Occupational Standards
– NASH-nuhl ok-yuh-PAY-shuhn-uhl
STAN-duhdz – The Hairdressing and
Beauty Therapy Industry Authority
(Habia) writes the standards for the
hairdressing and beauty therapy
industries. Your N/SVQ is based on
standards written by Habia. You can
read these to check what you need
to be competent at in order to gain
your N/SVQ.

**National Vocational Qualification
(NVQ)** – NASH-nuhl vuh-KAY-shuhn-uhl
kwol-if-i-KAY-shuhn -- EN-VEE-KYOO –
A 'competence-based' qualification:
this means you carry out practical,
work-related tasks designed to help
you develop the skills and knowledge
to do a job effectively.

Natural daylight – NACH-ruhl DAY-liyt – Ideal for day make-up or bridal make-up application.

Natural nail overlay – NACH-ruhl NAYL OH-vuh-lay – Coating the nail with materials used in repairs or extensions to keep the nail strong. Used in nail enhancements.

Necessary actions – NESS-uh-serr-i AK-shuhnz – When a client is not suitable for the treatment and therefore it cannot be carried out, they would need to seek medical advice. In some instances the treatment could be modified.

Needle-stick injury – NEEDL-STIK IN-juh-ree – A type of injury where the therapist accidentally injures themselves with a used needle during electrical epilation.

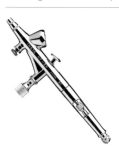

Needles – NEEDLZ – Sharp instrument in the centre of the airbrush down which the paint travels. This can also regulate the size of the spray.

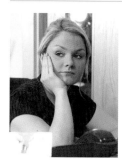

Negative attitude and behaviour – NEG-uh-tiv AT-it-yood uhnd bi-HAYV-ee-uh – This includes rudeness, bad temper, indifference, arrogance, poor timekeeping and closed body language.

Neuro-muscular – NYOO-roh-MUSS-kyuh-luh – A firm form of massage used to stimulate nerves.

New clients – NYOO KLIY-uhnts – Clients that are new to the salon and the therapist.

Non-conventional – NON-kuhn-VEN-shuhn-uhl – Something not normally used.

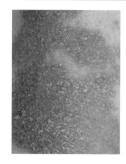

Non-infectious skin condition – NON-in-FEK-shuhss SKIN kun-DISH-uhn – A skin condition that does not spread from one person to another, for example eczema.

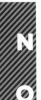

Non-verbal

Non-verbal – NON-VUR-buhl – Use of body language and writing to communicate with the client.

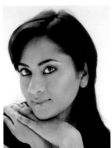

Normal hair
– NORM-uhl HAIR – Hair that is neither too dry nor too greasy.

Normal skin – NOR-muhl SKIN – An uncommon skin type with small pores and a smooth texture, an even colouring, and no blemishes, flaky or oily patches present.

Nozzle – NOZL – This keeps the needle in place and can also regulate the size of the spray.

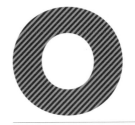

Objection/overcoming objections – uhb-JEK-shun/oh-vuh-KUM-ing uhb-JEK-shuhnz – An objection can be seen as the client putting up resistance to buying the product. A good sales person will be able to recognise if the objection is valid, and so close the discussion, or if the client just needs reassurance, in which case they will convince the client that they are doing the right thing by buying it.

Objectives – uhb-JEK-tivz – Your line manager will set you objectives that you need to achieve in a year. You should discuss short-term steps to help you achieve them.

Observation – ob-zuh-VAY-shuhn – To watch and receive knowledge information on what someone is achieving.

Obstruction – uhb-STRUK-shuhn – An item in the way of where you wish to get to, eg a blocked emergency door.

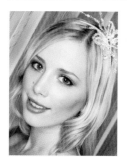

Occasion – uh-KAY-zhuhn – A special event (such as a wedding or party) for which clients often have their make-up done.

Occipital bone – ok-SIP-it-uhl BOHN – The bone across the back of the head above the nape area.

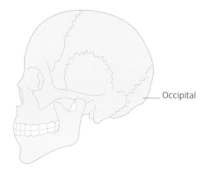

Occipital

Occupational role – ok-yuh-PAY-shuhn-uhl ROHL – The activities that a person is employed to carry out as part of their job.

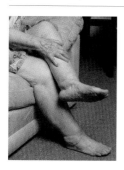

Oedema – i-DEE-muh – Swelling in the tissues due to a build-up of excess fluid. It is often referred to as water retention and is common in the feet and ankles.

Olfactory system – ol-FAK-tuh-ree SISS-tuhm – The system in the body that provides us with the sense of smell.

Oligomer – uh-LIG-uh-muh – Chains of monomers that are considerably shorter than a polymer.

One piece needle – WUN PEESS NEEDL – A needle made from a single piece of metal. It is used for hair removal methods of electrical epilation.

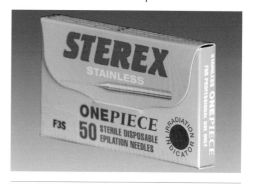

Onychia – o-NIK-ee-uh/oh-NIK-ee-uh – Bacterial infection that affects the nail folds, resulting in weeping and pus around the nail.

Onychocryptosis – on-i-koh-krip-TOH-siss – Commonly known as an ingrowing toenail, the nail grows into the skin at the side of the nail wall.

Onychogryphosis – on-i-koh-gri-FOH-siss – The nail plate enlarges, thickens and often curves. This usually occurs in older people.

Onycholysis – on-i-KOL-iss-iss – Separation of the nail plate from the nail bed.

Onychomadesis – ON-ik-oh-muh-DEE-siss – Severe separation of the nail plate from the nail bed, resulting in the nail falling off completely.

Onychomycosis – on-i-koh-miy-KOH-siss – A fungal infection of the nails, also referred to as tinea ungium.

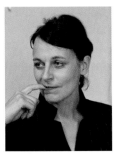

Onychophagy – on-i-KOF-uh-jee – The term used for nail biting.

Onychoptosis – ON-ik-oh-TOH-siss – Periodic shedding of part of, or the whole, nail.

Onychorrexis – on-i-kuh-REK-siss – Nails that are dry, split and brittle.

Open pores – OH-puhn PORZ – Small pin pricks on the surface of the skin, commonly found over the nose, chin and forehead. They may extend out over the cheeks. Open pores are a skin characteristic of an oily skin.

Open questions – OH-puhn KWESS-chuhnz – A questioning technique used to obtain more information, for example 'How would you like your make-up to look?' – the response has to include more detail than that of a closed question.

Optical brightener – OP-ti-kuhl BRIYT-nuh – This is added to nail products to make colours look brighter and to enhance the white products to make them look crisp, clean and bright.

Optional unit – OP-shuhn-uhl YOO-nit – Units that can be chosen by the candidate depending on the career direction of the student.

Oral hygiene – OR-uhl HIY-jeen – Regular cleaning of the teeth to ensure fresh breath and to prevent tooth decay.

Orbicularis oculi – or-bik-yuh-LAIR-iss OK-yuh-liy – Muscle that surrounds the eyes.

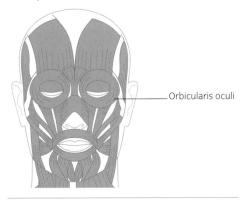

Orbicularis oculi

Orbicularis oris – or-bik-yuh-LAIR-iss OR-iss – Facial muscle that surrounds the mouth.

Organisational requirements – or-guhn-iy-ZAY-shuhn-uhl ruh-KWIY-uh-muhnts – Working practices and conditions specified by the salon.

Ornamentation – or-nuh-men-TAY-shuhn – An object used to complement a style, which adds interest and detail to the finished look.

Osteoporosis – OSS-tee-oh-por-ROH-siss – A disease in which the bones become extremely porous and are subject to fracture.

Otoplasty – OT-oh-plass-tee – The surgical repair, restoration or alteration of the external part of the ear.

Oval nail shape – OH-vuhl NAYL SHAYP – Where the sides of the free edge are curved to make the nail and finger appear longer and thinner.

Overexposure – OH-vuh-eks-POH-zhuh – Being regularly exposed to a product or chemical. You might not be allergic to the substance at first, but the body's immune system could develop sensitivity to it over time.

Overlay – OH-vuh-lay – The covering placed on the natural nail, or a natural nail with a tip in either liquid and powder, gel or wrap systems.

Oxidisation – ok-sid-iy-ZAY-shuhn – Occurs when tint colour is mixed with hydrogen peroxide, enabling the tint particles to swell and remain in the cortex of the hair. This gives the hair a permanent colour.

Oxygenating cream/serum – OK-si-jen-ay-ting KREEM/SEER-uhm – A product used with direct high frequency (DHF) to improve and enhance its effects.

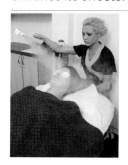

Ozone – OH-zohn – A gas produced when using direct high frequency – the current mixes with oxygen in the air. Ozone has a very distinct smell. It has a drying, antibacterial effect so it's ideal for problem and oily skins.

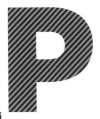

Pacemaker – PAYSS-may-kuh – An electrical device to stimulate and control the heart.

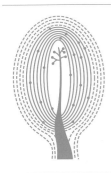

Pacinian corpuscles – puh-SIN-ee-uhn KOR-pusslz – Nerve endings that respond to pressure and are found deep in the reticular region.

Palatine – PAL-uh-tiyn/PAL-uh-tin – Two bones forming the floor of the nose and the roof of the mouth.

Palette – PAL-it – A board on which the artist dispenses and mixes colours.

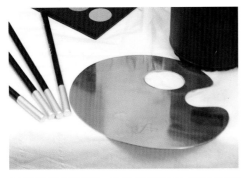

Palmaris longus – pal-MAH-riss/pal-MA-riss LONG-guss – Muscle that lies between the flexor carpi ulnaris and flexor carpi radialis. Flexes the wrist.

Pancake – PAN-kayk – Invented by Max Factor in the 1930s to replace greasepaint, this is a thick, densely pigmented full-coverage base.

Papule – PAP-yool – A hard red spot which does not contain pus and is often very painful.

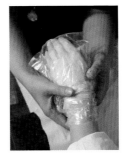

Paraffin wax treatment – PARR-uh-fin WAKS TREET-muhnt – Covering the hands in a warm paraffin wax liquid, building up several layers to retain the heat and wrapping in towels for a period of time. This will moisturise, soften and nourish the hands.

Parasite – PARR-uh-SIYT – An organism that lives in close relationship with another organism, causing it harm. For example, viruses are common parasites. The parasite has to be in its host to live, grow and multiply.

Parasitic infection – parr-uh-SIT-ik in-FEK-shuhn – Insect or animal parasites that either live on the hair of the skin or may even burrow under the skin. It is very contagious.

Parietal – puh-RIY-uh-tuhl – Two bones that form the crown of the skull.

Paronychia – parr-uh-NIK-ee-uh – A bacterial infection of the nail wall or cuticle. Symptoms include pain, swelling, redness and, in severe cases, pus.

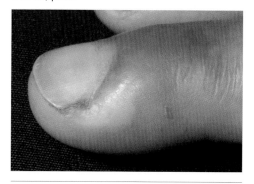

Parotid – puh-ROH-tid – Lymph node found just in front of the ear.

Passive electrode – PASS-iv i-LEK-trohd – Sometimes referred to as a non-working electrode, this is used in facial or body electrical treatments. The electrode is either given to the client to hold or placed on the skin to complete the electrical current flow.

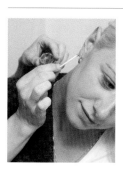

Patch test – PACH test – A test carried out 24 hours before the treatment to see if the client is allergic to the tinting products.

Patella – puh-TEL-uh – More commonly known as the kneecap.

Pathogens – PATH-uh-juhnz – Also known as an infectious agent or germ, it is an agent that causes damage to its host. There are different types, for example viral, bacterial and fungal. Bacteria that cause disease are called pathogenic bacteria.

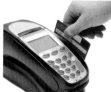

Payment card – PAY-muhnt KAHD – This refers to a debit or credit card.

Payment discrepancies – PAY-muhnt diss-KREP-uhn-siz – When a payment can't be made. Reasons for this may be an invalid credit/debit card or a fraudulent card.

Payment dispute – PAY-muhnt diss-PYOOT – When there is a problem with a payment, for example an invalid debit/credit card, or if you suspect the card is fraudulent.

Payment methods – PAY-muhnt METH-uhdz – These may include cash, credit/debit cards, cheque or cash alternatives (for example, vouchers).

Pectoralis – pek-tuh-RAY-liss/pek-tuh-RA-liss – Muscle that extends over the chest, attaching at the top of the arm.

Pediculosis capitis – pi-dik-yuh-LOH-siss kuh-PIY-tiss – This condition is caused by an infestation of the head by lice. The head louse (pediculus humanus capitis) attacks the skin and feeds by puncturing the skin to suck the blood; it lays eggs (ova) on the hair close to the skin. The symptoms are an itchy scalp and red areas; you should recommend treatment by a doctor or products from a chemist.

Pedicure – PED-i-kyoo-uh – Treatments applied to improve the appearance of the feet.

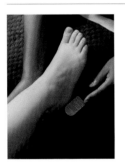

Pedicure tools – PED-i-kyoo-uh TOOLZ – A variety of tools used during a pedicure to reduce nail length, carry out cuticle work and remove hard skin.

Peer – PEER – Someone of the same rank or position as you.

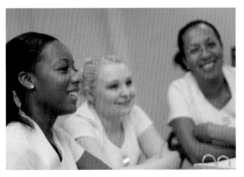

Peer assessment – PEER uh-SESS-muhnt – When a student's work is judged by another student at the same level.

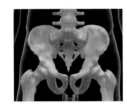

Pelvic girdle – PEL-vik GURDL – This is made up of two pelvic bones that provide support for the legs. The pelvic girdle also protects the internal pelvic organs.

Penile warts – PEE-niyl WORTS. N.B. 'warts' rhymes with 'forts' – Small, irregular cauliflower-like growths on the penis.

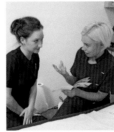

Performance appraisal – puh-FOR-muhnss uh-PRAY-zuhl – This is a method by which the job performance of an employee is evaluated (generally in terms of quality, quantity, cost and time) and it is carried out by a manager or supervisor.

Perionychium – perr-ee-oh-NIK-ee-uhm – The whole area surrounding the nail, from the nail wall on one side round to the nail wall on the other side.

Perm lotion – PURM LOH-shuhn – A chemical, usually thioglycolate, that when applied to the lashes will soften and break down the disulphide bonds, allowing the hair to bend into a new shape.

Perm rods – PURM RODZ – Cylindrical foam rods that come in various sizes and are used to curl the eyelashes.

Person specification – PUR-suhn spess-if-i-KAY-shuhn – Your role in the team and how you contribute to the team's effectiveness.

Personal development – PUR-suhn-uhl di-VEL-uhp-muhnt – Taking opportunities to develop your career and learn new skills.

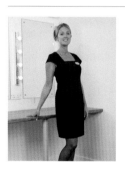

Personal hygiene – PUR-suhn-uhl HIY-jeen – Daily cleansing of the body, face, hands and feet, oral hygiene, and the use of skin and body care products.

Personal presentation – PUR-suhn-uhl prez-uhn-TAY-shuhn – The professional work-related appearance that is required in each establishment, eg hair is secured away from the face, and nails are clean, free of varnish and of a suitable length so as not to interfere with the treatment.

Personal Protective Equipment (PPE) – PUR-suhn-uhl pruh-TEK-tiv i-KWIP-muhnt -- PEE-PEE-EE – Relates to clothing and equipment to be used when carrying out services and includes the use of gloves and aprons when waxing to reduce the risk of cross-infection.

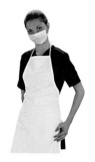

Personal Protective Equipment at Work Regulations – PUR-suhn-uhl pruh-TEK-tiv i-KWIP-muhnt uht WURK reg-yuh-LAY-shuhnz – When working with chemicals or products that may cause harm, it is the responsibility of the employer to provide personal protective equipment for the employee, who must use it.

Personal space – PUR-suhn-uhl SPAYSS – The space or 'aura' around a person. Many people feel uncomfortable if this space is invaded, so take care not to get too close, as appropriate to the situation. For example, you will obviously be touching your client's face while giving a facial, but that doesn't mean they'd be comfortable with you doing this in the reception area!

Personal survival budget – PUR-suhn-uhl suh-VIY-vuhl BUJ-it – The amount of money needed to maintain a reasonable and realistic lifestyle.

Personal targets – PUR-suhn-uhl TAH-gits – Individually agreed development and productivity goals for each staff member to work towards.

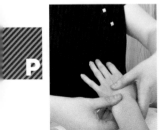

Petrissage – PET-ri-sahzh or pet-ri-SAHzh – A massage technique which applies alternating pressure to the tissues of the skin, lifting them away from the underlying structures.

pH – pee-AICH – The level of acidity and alkalinity measured on the pH scale, which goes from 0–14, with 7 being neutral: 0–6.9 is a low pH and is acid; 7.1–14 is a high pH and is alkaline. The skin's pH balance is between 4.5 and 6.2.

Phalanges – fuh-LAN-jeez – Fourteen individual bones that make up the fingers and toes.

Photo keratitis – FOH-toh kerr-uh-TIY-tiss – A corneal burn caused by UVB rays. The eyes become itchy and light sensitive.

Photographer's assistant – fuh-TOG-ruf-uhz uh-SISS-tuhnt – The person responsible for setting up, holding the reflectors, taking light readings and looking after the camera equipment.

Photosensitivity – foh-toh-senss-i-TIV-it-ee – A chemical or electrical reaction to light.

Phototoxicity – foh-toh-tok-SISS-it-ee – The effect certain oils have of making the skin more sensitive in the presence of sunlight.

Physiological effects – fiz-ee-uh-LOJ-ikl i-FEKTS – The effects that the oils have on the systems of the body.

Pilosebaceous unit – PIY-loh-suh-BAY-shuhs YOO-nit – A unit made up of the hair follicle, sebaceous gland, arrector pili muscle and hair shaft.

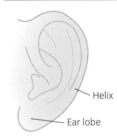

Helix

Ear lobe

Pinna – PIN-uh – The bulk of the ear. This is made up of cartilage and cartilaginous tissue so it can be moved around.

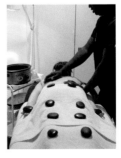

Placement – PLAYSS-muhnt – Either hot or cold stones are placed on the body, often on the Chakra points.

Plan for creating an image – PLAN fuh kree-AY-ting uhn IM-ij – The plan for creating an image will include making a design plan and producing a storyboard or mood board.

Planning – PLAN-ing – It is crucial that you carry out good planning before a photo shoot, hair show or other event. Poor planning results in poor performance.

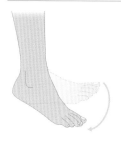

Plantar flexion – PLAN-tuh or PLAN-tah FLEK-shuhn – Anatomical term which describes the increase of the angle between the toes and the legs, eg pointing the toe downwards.

Planting the seed – PLAHN-ting dhuh SEED – Telling your client about the benefits of a product when you're discussing a treatment plan so that they'll be thinking about it throughout the treatment.

Platysma – pluh-TIZ-muh – Muscle that extends from the chin to the chest. It pulls the jaw and lower lip downwards.

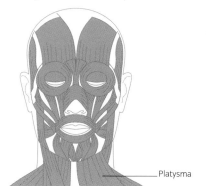

Platysma

Playboy – PLAY-boy – A term used within intimate female waxing. All hair is removed other than a pencil-wide strip over the pubic mound.

Point of sale (POS) – POYNT uhv SAYL -- PEE OH ESS – Usually the location where the credit/debit card transaction is processed, with the customer present. POS is also used as a broad term to describe the location where something is purchased.

Pointed nail shape – POYN-tid NAYL shayp – Where the free edge is shaped to a point. This places pressure on the sides, weakens the nail and makes it prone to breaking. This is the weakest of all nail shapes.

Policies and procedures – POL-uh-siz uhnd pruh-SEED-yuhz – Employers have these in place to protect you: they cover personal presentation, safe working and what to do in an emergency.

Polite manner – puh-LIYT MAN-uh – It's always crucial to adopt a polite manner when dealing with clients, which includes smiling, and saying 'please' and 'thank you'. Clients are more likely to return to the salon if they have been politely treated.

Polymer – POL-im-uh – A substance (eg a plastic) that is formed from many repeating smaller units.

Polymerisation – pol-im-uh-riy-ZAY-shuhn – The chemical process that turns a liquid (or semi-solid) into a solid.

Popliteal – pop-LIT-ee-uhl – Lymph nodes found at the back of the knee.

Porous – POR-ruhss – Absorbs liquid.

Portfolio – port-FOH-lee-oh – A collection of your work that could include log book photographs, sketches and testimonials from satisfied clients.

Positive attitude – POZ-it-iv AT-it-yood – Demonstrated with good body language, making eye contact, smiling and tone of voice.

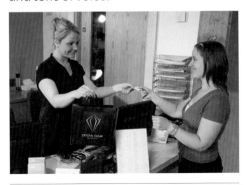

Positive body language – POZ-it-iv BO-dee LANG-gwij – Non-spoken communication such as posture, gesture or facial expression. An example of positive body language is smiling and looking at the person talking to you.

Positive image – POZ-it-iv IM-ij – In order to create a positive image at the reception, you must consider your personal appearance and behaviour, give efficient reception service, ensure a clean and tidy reception and display area, and meet and greet clients appropriately.

Positive impression – POZ-it-iv im-PRESH-uhn – Presenting a good image of yourself and your salon. Satisfied clients are more likely to return to the salon, so it's really important to give a positive impression.

Post-auricular – POHST-or-RIK-yuh-luh – Lymph node found behind the top of the ear.

Post-treatment – POHST-TREET-muhnt – What should happen after treatment, eg advice or necessary restrictions to activities.

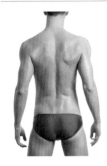

Posterior – poss-TEER-ee-uh – The back surface or back of the body.

Posture – POSS-chuh – The characteristic way in which a person holds their body.

Potentially infectious condition –
puh-TEN-shuh-lee in-FEK-shuhss kuhn-
DISH-uhn – A condition that may cause
visible signs of swelling, or redness on
the skin, and may spread, eg bacteria,
viruses or fungi.

Powder – POW-duh – Loose or
compact make-up that sets foundation,
disguises minor blemishes and makes
the skin appear oil-free and smooth.

Power jet massager – POW-uh JET
MASS-ah-zhuh or muh-SAH-zhuh – The
application of a powerful water hose to
the client's body, usually up and down
the spine. The client can stand or sit.

Pre-auricular – PREE-or-RIK-yuh-luh –
Lymph node found in front of the top of
the ear.

Pre-blended aromatherapy oils –
PREE-BLEN-did uh-ROH-muh-THERR-uh-
pee OYLZ – Essential oils that have been
pre-mixed with a vegetable oil base to
achieve specific effects, eg relaxation.

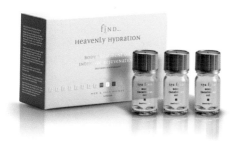

Pre-treatment – PREE-TREET-muhn –
Coating the cuticle with a polymer film,
which acts as a buffer to slow down the
chemical product.

Preparation of the client – prep-
uh-RAY-shuhn uhv dhuh KLIY-uhnt
– Procedures before treatment to
ensure the client is comfortable and
that the service can be given without
unnecessary interruptions.

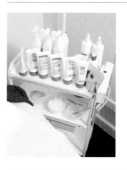

**Prepare the
work area**
– pri-PAIR dhuh
WURK AIR-ee-uh
– Arranging
products, tools
and equipment
ready for the
service to follow.

Presentation methods – prez-uhn-
TAY-shuhn METH-uhdz – Methods used
to explain concepts and ideas, such as
a short talk using Powerpoint slides.

Presentation/sales presentation
– prez-uhn-TAY-shuhn/SAYLZ prez-uhn-
TAY-shuhn – The process of explaining
the product or service to the client,
ideally including the product's features,
advantages and benefits.

Presenting a created image –
pri-ZEN-ting uh kree-AY-tid IM-ij –
You can present an image as part of
a show, a competition, a presentation
or a photographic shoot.

Pressure points – PRESH-uh POYNTS – Specific points on the body which, when stimulated, help to unblock energy flow.

Prices Act – PRIY-siz akt – The law that deals with how goods are priced and marked.

Prickle cells – PRIKL SELZ – A cell in the germinal layer of the skin.

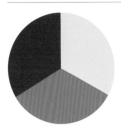

Primary colours – PRIY-muh-ree KUH-luhz – Every colour is made from a combination of red, yellow or blue. These three colours are known as the primary colours.

Procerus – proh-SEER-uhss – Muscle that runs from the brow to the nasal bone.

Product and Treatment Liability – PROD-uhkt uhnd TREET-muhnt liy-uh-BIL-it-ee – Insurance that protects salons against claims for injury or damage caused by treatments, services or products.

Productivity – prod-uhk-TIV-it-ee – The amount of work you do. If you work effectively, you will be highly productive.

Professional advice – pruh-FESH-uh-nuhl uhd-VYSS – Giving advice to a person based on your skills, knowledge and professional experiences.

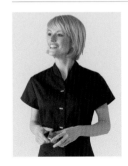

Professional image – pruh-FESH-uh-nuhl-IM-ij – Presenting yourself well in the salon, including following the rules of the dress code and using positive body language.

Professional indemnity insurance – pruh-FESH-uh-nuhl in-DEM-nit-ee in-SHOR-ruhnss – This will cover the salon against damages: for example, a customer might claim damages if their scalp is burned by incorrectly mixed chemicals.

Professionalism – pruh-FESH-uh-nuhl-izm – The codes of conduct and behaviour that you must follow within a job role, and the behaviour expected by clients and colleagues.

Profit and loss – PROF-it uhnd LOSS – A financial statement that summarises the financial transactions for a business over a period in time.

Prominent and protruding –
PROM-in-uhnt uhnd pruh-TROO-ding –
Sticking out.

Promotions – pruh-MOH-shuhnz
– Ways of informing the client about
products or services to increase
interest and, if relevant, sales.

Prone – PROHN – Lying face down.

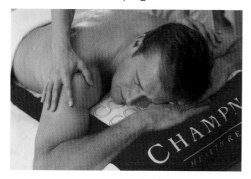

Props – PROPS – Items used as part
of a photo shoot to add interest and
support the theme.

**Provision and use of work
equipment regulations** – pruh-
VIZH-uhn uhnd YOOSS uhv WURK
i-KWIP-mhnt reg-yuh-LAY-shuhnz –
Employers must ensure that all who use
the equipment have been adequately
trained. You must ensure that you
are competent when using tools and
equipment in the salon.

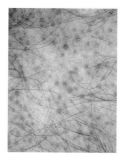

Pseudofolliculitis
– SYOO-doh
fo-lik-yoo-LIY-tiss
– This can develop
after waxing.
The hairs become
distorted and
grow back
into the follicle,
causing inflamed pustules that
can become infected.

PSI – PEE-ESS-IY – Pounds per square
inch is a measurement of the amount
of pressure put out by an airbrush. A
higher PSI will produce a heavier result,
while a low PSI will create a sheer finish.

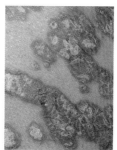

Psoriasis –
suh-RIY-uh-siss
– A chronic
inflammation.
Symptoms include
patches of itchy,
red and flaky skin.
This skin may
also be covered
with silvery or
white scales.

Psychological effects – siy-kuh-
LOJ-ikl i-FEKTS – The effects that
essential oils have on the mind,
memory and instincts.

Pterygium – terr-IJ-ee-uhm – Overgrowth of the cuticle, sometimes covering the whole of the nail plate, particularly if the nail is tiny, for example the little toenail.

Public Liability Insurance – PUB-lik liy-uh-BIL-it-ee in-SHOR-ruhnss – Protects the business financially from accidental injury to a client or member of the public, or from damage to their property.

Pulmonary circulation – PUL-muh-nuh-ree sirk-yuh-LAY-shuhn – The section of the blood circulatory system that involves the heart and the lungs.

Pulsing – PUL-sing – When the air is interrupted from travelling through the airbrush; this is useful to produce differing textured effects.

Purchaser – PUR-chiss-uh – Someone who buys a product.

Pustule – PUSS-tyool – An inflamed spot which contains pus.

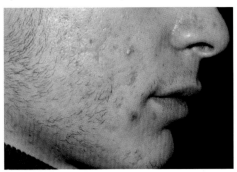

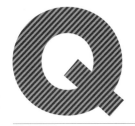

Quadratus labii superioris – kwod-RAY-tuhss/kwod-RAH-tuhss LAY-bee soo-PEER-ree-OR-riss – Facial muscle which forms expressions.

Quadratus lumborum – kwod-RAY-tuhss/kwod-RAH-tuhss lum-BOR-ruhm – A muscle found in the lower back. It runs from the lower ribs to the pelvis and helps flex the spine laterally.

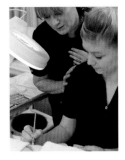

Quality management – KWOL-it-ee MAN-ij-muhnt – The implementation of effective systems and procedures relating to tasks carried out each day in the salon.

Questioning – KWES-chuh-ning – Open questions are used when you need to gain information and need to keep a conversation going, eg who, what, when, how. Closed questions are used when you wish to summarise and move on; they will be answered by yes or no.

Questionnaire – kwess-chuh-NAIR – A method of collecting feedback from clients to be used for evaluation purposes.

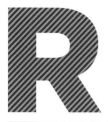

R

Race Relations Act – RAYSS ri-LAY-shuhnz akt – Protects people from discrimination on the grounds of colour, race, nationality or ethnic origins.

Radiotherapy – RAY-dee-oh-THERR-uh-pee – A treatment used to reduce cancerous tumours.

Radius – RAY-dee-uhss – Bone located in the middle of the forearm.

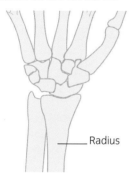

Radius

Rapport – ra-POR – A relationship of understanding, trust and agreement between two or more people.

Rebalance – ree-BAL-uhnss – A rebalance is carried out in nail enhancements, usually every four weeks. All three zones of the nail are redefined and the overlay is replaced.

Rebookings – ree-BUUK-ingz – Clients who remain loyal to the salon but are happy to see any therapist.

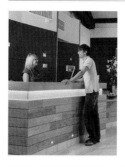

Reception – ri-SEP-shuhn – The area where clients book and make payments for services.

Reception stationery – ri-SEP-shuhn STAY-shun-uh-ree – Writing materials such as pencils, rubbers, message pads and appointment cards.

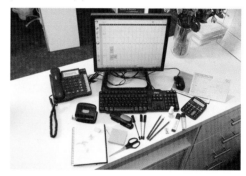

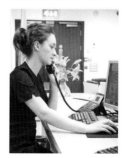

Receptionist – ri-SEP-shuhn-ist – In a salon or spa, this person greets clients and also makes the appointments for the services and treatments being carried out. They may also be responsible for answering any enquiries made by clients.

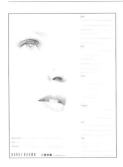

Record card – REK-ord KAHD – Contains information about each client, including the date and details of each treatment received, and products purchased.

Rectus abdominus – REK-tuhss ab-DOM-i-nuhss – Muscle found on the anterior abdomen. It flexes the trunk.

Rectus femoris – REK-tuhss FEM-uh-riss – One of the muscles that form part of the group called the quadriceps. It runs from the pelvis down the front of the leg to the tibia, and flexes the hip and extends the knee.

Reduction – ruh-DUK-shuhn – The chemical process of softening the hair to shape it around the perm rod – the first stage of eyelash perming.

Referral – ri-FUR-ruhl – When a client is advised to seek further advice on something from a person more knowledgeable in the subject; for example if a client had visible signs of headlice, you would refer them to a pharmacist.

Refractive index – ri-FRAK-tiv IN-deks – The speed at which light passes through a substance.

Regrowth – ree-GROHTH – The hair growth following a hair removal service.

Regulations – reg-yuh-LAY-shuhnz – Rules that must be followed, by law.

Relaxation room – ree-lak-SAY-shuhn room – A room of ambient temperature to induce relaxation.

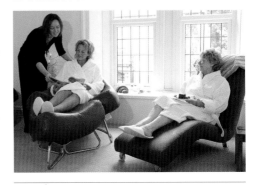

Relaxed pores – ruh-LAKST PORZ – When the walls of a pore have relaxed this causes the pore to appear larger than it is: a relaxed pore.

Relevant person – REL-uh-vuhnt PUR-suhn – A person who has set you the task and whose approval you will need to seek before commencing work, or a person who you will need to work together with to be able to complete the job.

Repair – ri-PAIR – A repair refers to a single nail enhancement, which may have been damaged before a maintenance service is due.

Repetitive Strain Injury (RSI) – ri-PET-uh-tiv STRAYN IN-juh-ree -- AH ESS IY – Injury resulting from doing one type of action too much. The wrist and fingers are especially prone to RSI.

Reporting of Injuries, Diseases and Dangerous Occurrences Regulations (RIDDOR) – ri-POR-ting uhv IN-juh-riz diz-EE-ziz unhd DAYN-juh-ruhss uh-KURR-uhn-siz reg-yuh-LAY-shuhnz (RID-or) – If you or your client suffer from personal injury at work then it must be reported in the salon accident book. This is to inform the employer and so that serious injury may be reported to the local enforcement officer.

Resale Price Act – REE-sayl PRYS akt – This act prevents manufacturers from imposing a specified retail price for goods. It is unlawful for a supplier to impose a minimum retail price by withholding supplies of the goods or discriminating in any other way. Many companies do however have a recommended retail price which they suggest their customers use.

Resin – REZ-in – An adhesive used in the wrap system. It can also be an ingredient found in a pigment stick.

Resources – ruh-ZOR-siz – The requirements for an activity. They include people, equipment, time, facilities and other things used to plan and carry it out.

Respiratory problems – ruh-SPI-ruh-tree PROB-luhmz – Breathing problems.

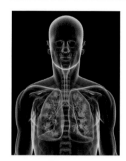

Respiratory system – ruh-SPI-ruh-tree SISS-tuhm – The breathing in and out of air, and using this air in the body.

Responsibilities – ruh-spon-suh-BIL-it-eez – The duties that a person within a particular job role is expected to perform.

Responsible person – ruh-SPON-sibl PUR-suhn – A person allocated with the responsibility of dealing with hazards and risks as they arise. This can be the salon owner, manager, a senior therapist, or a designated health and safety manager.

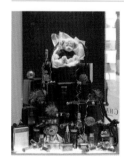

Retail displays – REE-tayl diss-PLAYZ – A colourful, clean, tidy and eye-catching display of all the products and tools that are available for sale to the clients.

Retin A – RET-in AY – A topical cream derived from vitamin A, prescribed for its anti-ageing effects or the treatment of moderate acne. As it thins the skin, it is a contra-indication to micro-dermabrasion.

Return clients

Return clients – ruh-TURN KLIY-uhnts – Clients that have returned to the same therapist and remain loyal to them.

Rhinoplasty – RIYN-oh-plast-ee – The technical name for a 'nose job'.

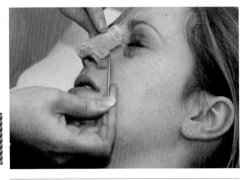

Rhytidectomy – rit-uh-DEK-tuh-mee – The technical name for a facelift.

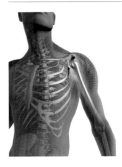

Ribs – RIBZ – Twelve pairs of ribs that form the protective thoracic cage.

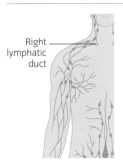

Right lymphatic duct

Right lymphatic duct – RIYT lim-FAT-ik DUKT – Lymph nodes found at the base of the neck on the right. It drains waste from the right side of the head, the right arm and the right side of the torso.

Ringworm – RING-wurm – (also known as Tinea) a contagious fungal infection where there are circles of red itchy skin, which heal from the centre. Can be found on the skin, nails or scalp.

Risk – RISK – The likelihood of a hazard occurring, eg if the wires on your equipment are frayed there is a greater risk of electric shocks.

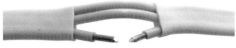

Risk assessment – RISK uh-SESS-muhnt – An assessment of all the possible hazards in a business, including their location and whether they are a high or low risk. The assessment also includes suggestions on how these risks can be controlled, managed or eliminated.

Risorius – ri-SOR-ree-uhss/ri-ZOR-ree-uhss – Muscle that runs from the corners of the mouth.

Role – ROHL – The actions and activities expected of a person within a particular job.

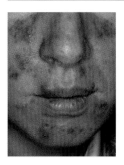

Rosacea – roh-ZAY-shee-uh – Chronic inflammation of the skin producing a characteristic red butterfly effect with pustules and papules, but no comedones.

Rosin – ROZ-in – An ingredient often found in wax, which would contra-indicate wax treatment if the client is allergic to sticking plasters, of which it is a component.

Round nail shape – ROWND NAYL SHAYP – Where the free edge is rounded. An ideal shape for short and bitten nails.

RPM – AH-PEE-EM – Revolutions per minute, indicated on compressor machines.

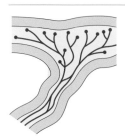

Ruffini corpuscles – ru-FEE-nee KOR-pusslz – Nerve endings that respond to heat and are found deep in the papillary region.

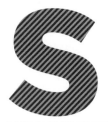

Sable brush – SAYBL BRUSH – A make-up brush made out of horse hair.

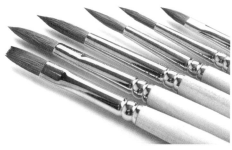

R

S

Safe and hygienic working practices – SAYF uhnd hiy-JEE-nik WUR-king PRAK-tiss-iz – To work safely and hygienically in the salon, you must use the PPE provided, follow COSHH, use appropriate methods of sterilisation, and follow the relevant health and safety legislation.

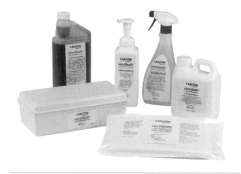

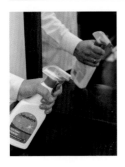

Safe working methods – SAYF WUR-king METH-uhdz – Working in a way that will not increase the risk of someone in your workplace being injured.

Safety considerations – SAYF-tee kuhn-sid-uh-RAY-shuhnz – You need to ensure that you carry out the right preparation, follow COSHH, use safe working methods, use or wear your provided PPE and follow the manufacturer's instructions when using products or equipment.

Safety Data Sheet – SAYF-tee DAY-tuh SHEET – Provides information on chemical products that helps users of those chemicals to make a risk assessment. It describes the hazards the chemical presents and gives information on handling, storage and emergency measures in case of an accident.

Sale and Supply of Goods Act – SAYL uhnd suh-PLIY uhv GUUDZ akt – Legislation stating that goods sold must be as described, of suitable quality and fit for their intended purpose.

Sales forecast – SAYLZ FOR-kahst – Prediction of the future sales of a particular product, including treatments over a specific period of time based on past performance of the product, inflation rates, unemployment, consumer spending patterns, market trends and interest rates.

Sales techniques – SALYZ tek-NEEKS – Ways in which you will help the client to decide the product or service that will suit their needs.

Salon and legal requirements – SAL-o(ng) or suh-LO(ng) uhnd LEE-guhl ruh-KWY-uh-muhnts – Beauty therapy work rules and laws, issued by the salon management and government. These rules affect the salon and its day-to-day operation.

Salon junior – SAL-o(ng) or suh-LO(ng) JOO-nee-uh – A person who is employed to help the senior members of staff in a salon or spa. Their duties will include preparing the work area for a beauty treatment.

Salon manager – SAL-o(ng) or suh-LO(ng) MAN-i-juh – This person is in charge of the day-to-day running of the salon, for example making decisions on staff responsibilities and recruitment of employees.

S

Salon owner – SAL-o(ng) or suh-LO(ng) OH-nuh – A person who owns a salon business and makes important decisions regarding the overall running of the salon.

Salon policy – SAL-o(ng) or suh-LO(ng) POL-i-see – The procedures and requirements for salon processes and systems, for example staff grievances or client refunds.

Salon procedures – SAL-o(ng) or suh-LO(ng) pruh-SEED-yuhz – The rules and systems that your salon has in place. Your supervisor will inform you of these.

Salon requirements – SAL-o(ng) or suh-LO(ng) ruh-KWIY-uh-muhnts – The rules and regulations issued by the salon manager.

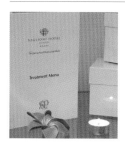

Salon services – SAL-o(ng) or suh-LO(ng) SUR-viss-iz – The services that are offered by the salon.

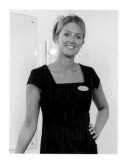

Salon standards for appearance and behaviour – SAL-o(ng) or suh-LO(ng) STAN-duhdz fuhrr uh-PEER-ruhnss uhnd bi-HAY-vee-uh – Your manager will show you how he/she expects you to dress and behave. There may be a dress code/uniform and a code of conduct, which states how you should look and behave.

Sanding bands – SAN-ding BANDZ – A disposable ring of sand paper, available in various grits. Used in nail enhancements.

Sanitisation – san-it-iy-ZAY-shuhn – The equipment you use should be in a hygienic condition before use, which means sanitising and sterilising it. Methods of doing this include using a UV cabinet.

Saponification – suh-pon-if-i-KAY-shuhn – An effect of the cathode as the active electrode in desincrustation causes the alkaline reaction to break down and soften the hardened sebum, creating a soaping effect.

Sartorius – sah-TOR-ree-uhss – Muscle that crosses the front of the thigh, from the outer side down to the inner side. It has many actions, including flexion and abduction of the thigh and flexion of the knee.

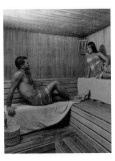

Sauna – SOR-nuh or SOW-nuh – A treatment room of timber construction where the air is heated to produce a therapeutic effect or, if infrared is used, the body is heated directly through infrared radiators in the sauna.

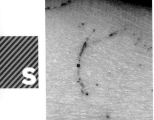

Scabies – SKAY-beez – This condition is caused by a reaction to an itch mite. The tiny animal parasite (sarcoptes scabiei) burrows through the skin and lays its eggs. The areas affected become extremely itchy, especially at night. There are reddish spots and burrows (greyish lines) under the skin. Refer sufferers to a doctor.

Scaling – SKAY-ling – The build-up of limescale and bacteria on a surface caused by water.

Scalp – SKALP – The top part of the head where the hair is located – on some people it is fairly flexible, while on others it is quite tight and rigid.

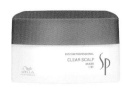

Scalp products – SKALP PRODuhkts – Products designed to be used on the head, which may be for the hair or the skin – these may stimulate the blood supply, soften the hair or cool the area, for example.

Scapula – SKAP-yuu-liy/SKAP-yuu-lee – More commonly known as a shoulder blade.

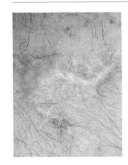

Scar tissue – SKAH TISH-yoo – Healed area where the skin is often a different colour; it may be red-looking and raised.

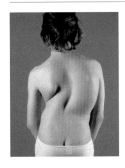

Scoliosis – skoh-lee-OH-siss or skol-ee-OH-siss – A sideways curvature to the spine, which can result in uneven hip and shoulder height.

Scrotum – SKROH-tuhm – A muscular sac that contains the testes.

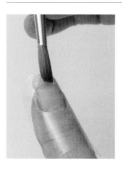

Sculptured nail – SKULP-chuhd NAYL – This nail enhancement technique extends the nail plate by building it onto a nail form.

Seasonal Affective Disorder (SAD) – SEEZ-uhn-uhl uh-FEK-tiv diss-OR-duh -- ESS-AY-DEE – A form of depressive illness only occurring during winter months, which is related to lack of sunshine and is responsive to phototherapy.

Seasonal offer – SEEZ-uhn-uhl OF-uh – Something that relates to the season, eg waxing is ideal for spring and summer to prepare for holidays and the warmer weather, whereas fake tans are good for the festive season, when people have parties to dress up for.

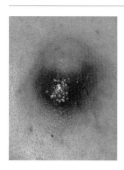

Sebaceous cyst – si-BAY-shuhss SIST – A lump of fibrous tissues and fluids. The most common sites for sebaceous cysts are the scalp, back and face.

Sebaceous gland – si-BAY-shuss GLAND – This gland is attached to the hair follicle in the skin and produces sebum, which is the skin's own natural moisture.

Seborrhoea – seb-uh-REE-uh – Excessively oily skin.

Sebum – SEE-buhm – Produced in the sebaceous gland and is the skin's own lubricant.

Secondary colours – SEK-uhn-dree KUH-luhz – Violet, orange and green.

Secretion – suh-KREE-shuhn – The release of a substance from a cell or gland.

Self-assessment – self-uh-SESS-muhnt – Students making judgments about their own work.

Semi-precious stones – SEM-ee-PRESH-uhss STOHNZ – Examples are quartz, topaz and carnelian. These stones are generally used as placement stones in stone therapy treatments.

Sensitive skin – SEN-sit-iv SKIN – Skin which reacts readily to products, heat or pressure. Whilst it can occur on any skin type, it usually has a fine texture, thin epidermis and blood vessels very close to the surface, which can result in blotchiness, redness, flushing, increased warmth and irritation if stimulated.

Sensory nerve endings – SEN-suh-ree NURV END-ingz – Found in the dermis, there are five types of sensory nerve endings: touch, pain, pressure and temperature.

Sepsis – SEP-siss – The presence of bacteria.

Serratus anterior – suh-RAY-tuhss/ suh-RAH-tuhss an-TEER-ree-uh – Muscle found around the side of the ribcage, under the arm. It helps to bring the scapula forwards.

Service plan – SUR-viss PLAN – A record of services performed, the outcomes and recommendations given.

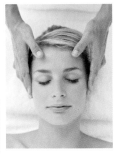

Services – SUR-viss-iz – The different types of beauty treatments offered to clients in salons, such as Indian head massage and camouflage make-up.

Sesame oil – SESS-uh-mee OYL – Used in Indian Head massage. Popular in Ayurveda, it has a high mineral content and so is useful for nourishing the hair.

Sex Discrimination Act – SEKS dis-krim-i-NAY-shuhn akt – Protects anyone against discrimination based on their sexuality.

Shader – SHAY-duh – A make-up product used to take attention away from a feature.

Shaping – SHAY-ping – A term used in intimate waxing to describe when a client requests a certain shape of hair in their pubic region. This shape is often achieved by using a stencil.

Sharps – SHAHPS – This term describes the blades used in safety razors. All blades should be disposed of in a yellow sharps container.

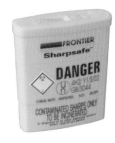

Sharps box – SHAHPS boks – The sharps box is where all used 'sharps' (ie blades) must be disposed of.

Showreel – SHOH-reel – A short DVD of your work to show to potential clients.

Shower – SHOW-uh – Used to cleanse the skin, regulate body temperature or as a spa treatment itself.

Side feed airbrush – SIYD feed AIR-brush – This is usually a larger cup attached to the side of the airbrush to hold paint.

Silicone-based make-up – SIL-i-kohn-BAYSST MAYK-up – Make-up which produces a fresh dewy look.

Single action airbrush – SING-guhl AK-shuhn AIR-brush – Like an aerosol, you press this down to get the paint.

Single action technique – SING-guhl AK-shuhn tek-NEEK – Derives its name from the fact that only one action is required for operation. The single action of depressing the trigger releases a fixed ratio of make-up to air gravity feed. The colour cup is on top of the brush.

Single follicle – SING-guhl FOL-ikl – A hair follicle only containing one hair shaft.

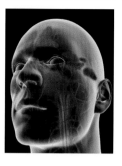

Sinuses – SIY-nuhsses-iz – There are four pairs of sinuses found in the face – frontal, sphenoid, ethmoidal and maxillary.

Siphon feed – SIY-fuhn FEED – The colour cup or container is either on the bottom or the side of the brush.

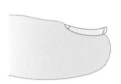

Ski jump nail – SKEE jump NAYL – A nail shape where the nail curves upwards from the cuticle to the free edge. A ski jump nail is also known as a spoon nail.

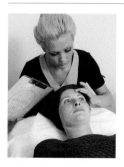

Skin analysis – SKIN uh-NAL-uh-siss – The process of closely looking at the client's skin after cleansing, using a magnifier with a light. This is an important part of the facial, as the findings are used to create a suitable treatment plan.

Skin blanching – SKIN BLAN-ching or BLAHN-ching – When the skin turns a white colour and swells. This occurs as a result of incorrect techniques when carrying out electrical epilation.

Skin characteristics – SKIN karr-ik-tuh-RISS-tiks – Typical features that indicate a skin type, eg open pores, shiny appearance and pustules are characteristics of an oily skin.

Skin colour – SKIN KUH-luh – The actual colour of the skin. This can range from very light to dark and can vary from area to area on one face.

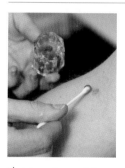

Skin sensitivity test – SKIN SEN-sit-iv-it-ee TEST – (sometimes referred to as a skin patch test) a test carried out 24 hours before the treatment to see if the client is allergic to certain products, eg tinting products and perming products.

Skin structure – SKIN STRUK-chuh
– The skin is the largest organ of the body. The skin has two main layers: the epidermis and dermis. Below these is a layer of subcutaneous fat.

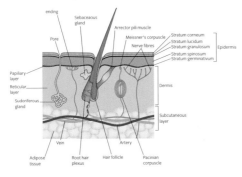

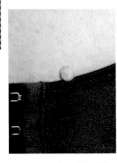

Skin tags – SKIN TAGZ – Also called papilloma or fibro-epithelial polyps. They are an overgrowth of epithelial tissue on a stalk, commonly found around the neck and axilla. They vary in size and colour.

Skin texture – SKIN TEKS-chuh –
A term used to refer to the thickness of the skin, which may be referred to as fine or coarse.

Skin type 1 – SKIN TIYP WUN – This is
very sensitive skin. Typically, the client has very pale skin, red/blonde hair and blue/green eyes.

Skin type 2 – SKIN TIYP TOO – This is
sensitive skin. Typically, the client has light to medium skin, fair to light brown hair and blue/green/grey eyes.

Skin type 3 – SKIN TIYP THREE – This
is normal skin sensitivity. Typically, the client has medium to olive skin, medium to brown hair and grey/brown eyes.

Skin type 4 – SKIN TIYP FOR – This skin
is very resistant to the sun. Typically, the client has dark olive to light brown skin, dark eyes and dark hair.

Skin types – SKIN TIYPS – Either dry
(lacking in oil), oily (excessive oil) or combination (a mixture of both).

Skin types 5 and 6 – SKIN TIYPS FIYV
uhnd SIKS – This is naturally tanned/dark skin. Typically, the client has dark hair and eyes.

Skin warming device – SKIN WOR-
ming di-VIYS N.B 'Warming' rhymes with 'forming' – Either an electrical facial steamer or hot damp towels. Both warm, cleanse, stimulate and soften the skin in preparation for extraction.

Sloughing – SLUF-ing – A term used
to describe the casting off of dead skin tissue.

Small Firms Enterprise Development Initiative – SMORL
FURMZ EN-tuh-priyz duh-VEL-uhp-muhnt in-ISH-uh-tiv – The leading organisation for small firms' development and support.

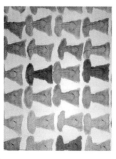

Small prosthetics – SMORL pross-THET-iks – Often made from silicone, these are 'false' noses, ear tips, chins and so on, which are applied and covered with make-up to blend in with the surrounding skin.

SMART targets – SMAHT TAH-gits – A management acronym to describe how targets should be written and planned: Specific, Measurable, Achievable, Realistic, Timebound.

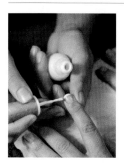

Smile line – SMIYL LIYN – The line that naturally occurs at the hyponychium – where the nail plate leaves the nail bed. It's called the smile line because it curves upwards like a smile.

Soft fat – SOFT FAT – Fat that feels wobbly and spongy to touch. Often found on the abdomen.

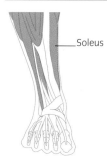

Soleus

Soleus – SOH-lee-uhss – Muscle that lies beneath the gastrocnemius and attaches to the Achilles tendon.

Solvents – SOL-vuhnts – Liquids that dissolve other solids. Nail polish remover is used to dissolve nail polish. The solvent keeps the polish in a liquid form until it evaporates and leaves behind the solid, dry polish.

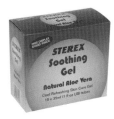

Soothing products – SOODH-ing PROD-uhkts – Products that are used on the skin following a waxing treatment to reduce any irritation, redness and minor swelling that might have occurred.

Sources of information (information methods) – SOR-siz uhv in-fuh-MAY-shuhn -- in-fuh-MAY-shuhn METH-uhdz – These include the internet, magazines, photographs, sketches, textbooks, television/DVDs, image libraries and hair/fashion shows.

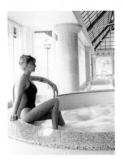

Spa – SPAH – The true meaning is a place that has naturally occurring mineral waters, such as Bath Spa or Leamington Spa in the UK. These are often hot when they come out through the earth.

Spa bath – SPAH BAHTH – This is often referred to as a jacuzzi or whirlpool. It has either circulating water or water forced through pipes to create a relaxing, bubbling effect.

Spa therapist – SPAH THERR-uh-pist – A therapist who specialises in spa treatments such as hydrotherapy and body wraps.

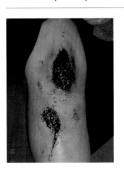

Special effects make-up – SPESH-uhl i-FEKTS MAYK-up – The creation of a look including wounds and injuries.

Specialist salons – SPESH-uh-list SAH-lo(ng)z or suh-LO(ng)z – Salons that specialise in certain services, for example male skin care, make-up for special occasions, etc.

Specialist skin care products – SPESH-uh-list SKIN KAIR PROD-uhkts – These are used to target specific skin improvement and include eye gels/creams, neck creams and lip products.

Sphenoid – SFEE-noyd – One bone forming the back of the eye sockets.

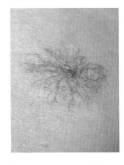

Spider naevi – SPIY-duh NEE-viy – This is usually a central small blood spot with thread veins, which radiates outwards.

Spillage – SPIL-ij – A product or substance that is dropped or leaked onto the floor.

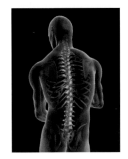

Spine – SPIYN – The spine is made up of seven cervical bones, 12 thoracic bones, five lumbar bones, five bones fused together to make up the sacrum and four bones fused together to make up the coccyx.

Spirit gum – SPIRR-it GUN – An adhesive solution made of gum (resin) and ether, and used to fix a variety of items to the skin, eg glitter and sequins. It is a potential allergen, so it is vital to perform a skin sensitivity test before use.

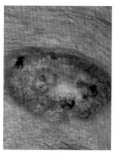

Squamous cell carcinoma – SKWAY-muhss SEL kah-si-NOH-muh – A form of skin cancer that affects the epidermal layers. It is characterised by ulcers on the skin that do not heal.

Square nail shape – SKWAIR NAYL SHAYP – Where the free edges is straight across and makes the sides sharp and prone to catching on things. This shape makes long nail beds and fingers appear shorter and fuller.

Squoval nail shape – SKWOH-vuhl NAYL SHAYP – Where the nail is straight across at the free edge with the sides rounded off. An ideal shape for short or bitten nails.

Staff induction – STAHF in-DUK-shuhn – A process to introduce new employees to their jobs and working environment.

Steam – STEEM – Water is heated to create steam, used for its therapeutic effect. This can be enjoyed individually in a steam bath or communally in a steam room.

Steam bath or cabinet – STEEM BAHTH or KAB-uh-nit – The client sits on a seat in a steam-infused cabinet, with their head popping up out of a hole in the top of the cabinet.

Steam room – STEEM room – A small room that is infused with steam. Many clients sit on marble slabs.

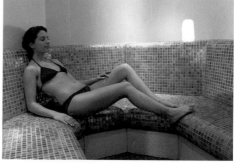

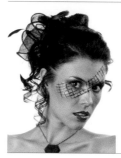

Stencil – STEN-suhl – A plastic sheet that has had pieces cut out of it, so paint can penetrate through to leave a pattern when airbrushing.

Stencilling – STEN-suh-ling – A make-up technique using a pre-cut or custom designed template to achieve sharp definition and/or continuity and consistency.

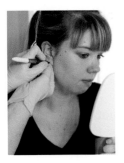

Sterile marker pen – STERR-iyl MAH-kuh pen – Used in ear piercing to mark the position for piercing on the ear lobes. The position is agreed with the client before the piercing takes place.

Sterilisation – sterr-il-iy-ZAY-shuhn – The process of destroying all micro-organisms and their spores.

Sterling – STUR-ling – This is the currency used in the UK and is also referred to as the 'Great British Pound' (GBP).

Sternocleidomastoid – STUR-noh KLIY-doh MAS-toyd – Muscle on the side of the neck that extends from below the ear to the sternum.

Sternum – STUR-nuhm – More commonly known as the breastbone.

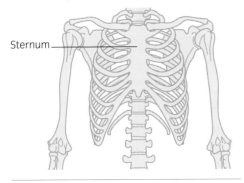

Sternum

Stock control – STOK kuhn-TROHL – The process of collecting information on supplies and equipment to allow the correct ordering to take place.

Stock control system – STOK kuhn-TROHL SISS-tuhm – A method of identifying stock levels and tracking stock for the purpose of efficient replenishment; it can be a manual or computerised system.

Stock rotation – STOK roh-TAY-shuhn – Placing new stock at the back of shelves, bringing the old stock forward to use first.

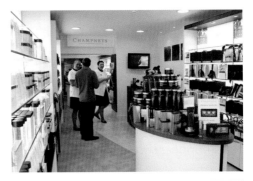

Stop point – STOP poynt – This is the part where the tip fits around the free edge of the natural nail plate.

Stratum corneum – STRAH-tuhm KOR-nee-uhm – Often referred to as the horny layer, the stratum corneum is the top outer layer of the epidermis. It is made up of dead, flattened, keratinised cells that are always being shed.

Stratum germinativum – STRAH-tuhm jur-min-uh-TIYV-uhm – Often referred to as the basal layer, the stratum germinativum is the bottom layer of the epidermis which attaches to the dermis. It is in this layer that new cells are formed by a process called mitosis.

Stratum granulosum – STRAH-tuhm gran-yoo-LOH-suhm – Often referred to as the granular layer, the stratum granulosum lies beneath the stratum lucidum. It is the layer where keratinisation is completed and the living skin cells are hardened and flattened.

Stratum lucidum – STRAH-tuhm LOO-sid-uhm – Often referred to as the clear layer, the stratum lucidum lies under the stratum corneum and is made up of tightly packed transparent cells. This layer is very thin on the face and thicker on the soles of the feet.

Stratum spinosum – STRAH-tuhm spin-OH-zuhm or spiyn-OH-zuhm – Often referred to as the prickle cell layer, the stratum spinosum lies beneath the stratum granulosum. The cells are rounded with spiky fingers that attach to other cells. This layer begins the keratinisation process.

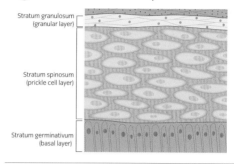

Stratum granulosum (granular layer)

Stratum spinosum (prickle cell layer)

Stratum germinativum (basal layer)

Strengths and weaknesses – STRENGTHS uhnd WEEK-niss-iz – Identify these in order to set targets. What are you good at? What do you feel that you need help with?

Stress area (or apex) – STRESS AIR-ee-uh or AY-peks – Also known as zone 2, this is where the overlay should be the thickest to ensure it is strong enough to resist breakage.

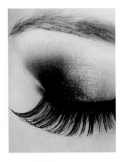

Strip lashes
– STRIP LASH-iz –
Available in pairs, these run the entire length of the eyelid and are applied to the skin just above the lash line. They are available in a variety of lengths, styles and thicknesses, and are designed to be removed nightly.

Striping pen – STRIY-ping pen –
A very fine brush used to make stripes or tapering stripes on the nail.

Structure of the skin – STRUK-chuh uhv dhuh SKIN – The skin is made up of the epidermis, dermis, subcutaneous layer, sweat glands, sebaceous glands and hair follicles.

Stye – STIY – A small boil at the base of the eyelash follicle which is red, sore and swollen.

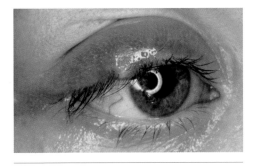

Sub-mandibular – sub man-DIB-yuh-luh – Lymph node found under the mandible.

Sub-mental – sub MEN-tuhl – Lymph node found under the chin.

Subcutaneous – sub-kyoo-TAY-nee-uhss – The layer found under the dermis, made up of adipose tissue (fat), which helps to protect the skin.

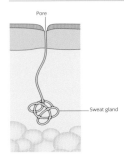

Sudoriferous gland – soo-duh-RIF-uh-ruhss or syoo-duh-RIF-uh-ruhss GLAND – (commonly known as the sweat gland). This excretes watery substances on to the surface of the skin.

Sugar paste – SHOOG-uh PAYST –
A mixture of ingredients (including sugar) which is heated to form a paste. This is applied with the hands in the direction of the hair growth, and removed against the hair growth with the hands in a swift action.

Sugar strip – SHOOG-uh STRIP –
A mixture of ingredients (including sugar) which is heated to form a paste. This is applied with either the hands or a spatula in the direction of the hair growth, and removed against the hair growth using either a paper or muslin strip pressed on the top.

Sun Protection Factor (SPF) – SUN pruh-TEK-shuhn FAK-tuh -- ESS-PEE-EF – Sun protection factor provides a certain amount of protection against UVB damage but not UVA damage.

Sunbed code of practice – SUN-bed KOHD uhv PRAK-tiss – A set of guidelines detailing the safe use of sunbeds.

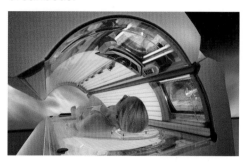

Sunburn – SUN-burn – Overexposure to UVB rays, resulting in inflamed, sore and red skin.

Superficial and deep cervical – soo-puh-FISH-uhl uhnd DEEP SUR-vikl – Lymph nodes found deep in the neck.

Superfluous hair – soo-PUR-floo-uhs HAIR – A general term used to describe any unwanted hair.

Superior – soo-PEER-ee-uh – In anatomy and physiology, this is when something is above or towards the top of the body, eg the head is superior to the spine.

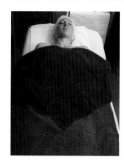

Supine – SOO-pyn – Lying face up.

Supplier – suh-PLIY-uh – Someone who supplies resources, equipment and materials.

Supra-clavicular – SOO-pruh kluh-VIK-yuh-luh – Lymph nodes of the head, found above the clavicle, just above the sternum.

Supra-trochlear – SOO-pruh TROK-lee-uh – Lymph nodes in the crease of the elbow and sometimes called cubital.

Suture – SOO-chuh – The point at which the bones of the skull are fused together.

Systemic circulation – siss-TEEM-ik or siss-TEM-ik sur-kyoo-LAY-shuhn – The blood circulatory system that involves the heart and rest of the body.

Systemic hair growth – siss-TEEM-ik or siss-TEM-ik HAIR GROHTH – Hormonal changes, either normal or abnormal, that may stimulate hair growth. Normal changes include puberty and the menopause; abnormal changes include Cushing's syndrome and polycystic ovary syndrome.

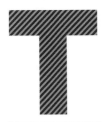

Tactile sensation – TAK-tiyl sen-SAY-shuhn – The sensation produced by pressure receptors in the skin.

Tan enhancer – TAN in-HAHN-suh – These include creams, gels, powders and illuminators, which are shimmery or bronzed to give a glowing look to the tan.

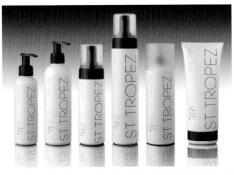

Tanning accelerator – TAN-ing uhk-SEL-uh-ray-tuh – Products designed to increase your body's natural production of melanin, thus increasing the effect of UV radiation on the skin. They can damage the skin and are not recommended.

Tapered nail shape – TAY-puhd NAYL SHAYP – Where the free edge becomes thinner towards the distal edge. Tapered nails are often the weakest nails but, if you don't file down the side walls, you shouldn't make the nail any weaker.

Tapotement/percussion – tuh-POHT-muhnt/puh-KUSH-uhn – Brisk movements are used in this technique in order to stimulate and tone the skin.

Tapping stones – TAP-ing stohnz – A technique used in stone therapy where one stone is held on the area and the other is used to tap on top of this stone.

Target – TAH-git – A task to complete (usually within a set timescale) to achieve a particular result. For example, you may be required to sell a number of services or products to meet your salon's sales targets or your own personal goal.

Target group – TAH-git GROOP – The clientele you are trying to attract into the salon. For example, a promotional activity to increase single eyelash extension treatments would probably be aimed at female clients.

Target setting – TAH-git SET-ing – You and your manager will spend some time discussing your training needs, which will be split into specific, measurable and achievable sections. Your achievement of these targets will be used to measure your progress.

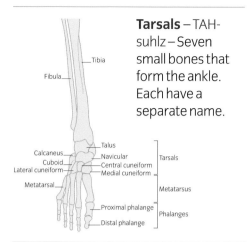

Tarsals – TAH-suhlz – Seven small bones that form the ankle. Each have a separate name.

Team – TEEM – A group of people who work together.

Team work – TEEM wurk – People working together effectively to achieve a particular aim.

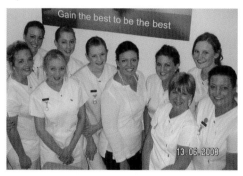

Gain the best to be the best

Techniques – tek-NEEKS – The different methods used to create the finished image, for example make-up techniques, application of false eyelashes, clothes and hair.

Telangiectasia – tel-an-jee-ek-TAY-see-uh – The technical term for thread veins, which are tiny red thread-like lines on the skin. Also known as dilated or broken capillaries.

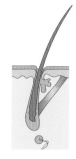

Telogen hair – TEE-loh-jen or TEL-oh-jen HAIR – The resting stage of the hair growth cycle, which can last for 3–4 months.

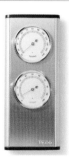

Temperature gauge – TEM-pruh-chuh GAYJ – Equipment used to measure temperature.

Temporal – TEM-pruhl – Two bones that form the sides of the cranium.

Temporalis – tem-puh-RA-liss/tem-puh-RAY-liss – Muscle on the side of the head that stretches to the mandible.

Temporary products – TEMP-puh-ruh-ree PROD-uhkts – Products that are not permanent and will fade, eg eyelash tint.

Tendon – TEN-duhn – Fibres that connect muscle to bone.

Tendonitis – ten-duhn-IY-tiss – Inflammation of a joint, often caused by overuse.

Tensor fasciae latae – TEN-suhh FASH-ee-iy LAH-tiy/FASH-ee-ee LAH-tee – Muscle that runs down the outer side of the thigh. It helps with flexion and abduction of the thigh.

Tepidarium – te-pi-DAIR-ee-um – A pleasant, warm relaxation room found in a spa.

Terminal hair – TUR-mi-nuhl HAIR – The eyebrows, eyelashes and scalp hair, as well as pubic hair.

Test patch – TEST pach – Either heat sensitive, thermal or tactile tests that are carried out to check the client's reaction to heat and the products used. Often used in waxing, facial electrical treatments and body electrical treatments.

Texturising materials – TEKS-chuh-riy-zing muh-TEER-ee-uhlz – In media make-up these include any product or ingredient that adds texture, such as fabric and gems.

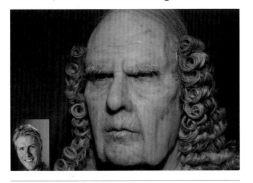

Thalassotherapy – thuh-lass-oh-THERR-uh-pee – The use of sea water in hydrotherapy treatments. Thalassotherapy spas are usually located near the sea.

The image – dhee IM-ij – The image is the total look. This includes hair make-up, clothes and jewellery. This can be avant-garde, based on a theme or a commercial look.

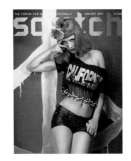

Theme – THEEM – A set outline, for example images reflecting an era or the front cover of a fashion magazine.

Thenar eminence – THEE-nuh EM-in-uhnss – This muscle is found in the palm of the hand at the base of the thumb. It controls the movement of the thumb.

Thermal and tactile tests – THUR-muhl uhnd TAK-tiyl TESTS – Tests that are carried out before using equipment on a client. Thermal tests check whether the client can tell hot from cold, while tactile tests focus on whether they can feel the difference between sharp and blunt.

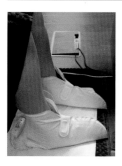

Thermal boots
– THUR-muhl
BOOTS – Heated
boots used to
speed up the
effects of foot
masks during
a pedicure.

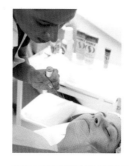

Threading
– THRED-ing –
A specialised
method of hair
removal using
the swift action
of fingers, thumbs
and tight thread.

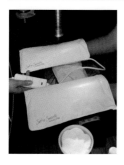

Thermal mitts
– THUR-muhl MITS
– Heated mitts
that are used to
speed up the
effects of a hand
mask during
a manicure.

Three-way stretch – THREE WAY
STRECH – A stretch technique used
in electrical epilation to maximise the
opening of the follicle. This makes the
insertion of the probe easier.

Tibia – TIB-ee-uh – More commonly
known as the shin bone.

Thermolysis – thur-MOL-iss-iss –
The destruction of tissues using heat,
eg in electrical epliation using short
wave diathermy.

Tibialis anterior – tib-ee-AL-iss/tib-
ee-AY-liss an-TEER-ee-uh – Muscle that
extends from the lateral edge of the
patella to the medial edge of the ankle.

Thoracic duct – thuh-RA-sik/thor-RA-
sik DUKT – Lymph nodes found beneath
the body of the sternum. Drains waste
from the left side of the head, the left
arm and the rest of the body.

Time management – TIYM MAN-ij-
muhnt – Organising your time well so
that you are as efficient as possible.
This can include planning ahead and
prioritising your tasks.

Thread – THRED – A loop of pure
cotton thread that is twisted and
used between the fingers to carry
out depilation.

Timebound – TIYM-bownd – An
activity or objective that has set dates
for tasks to be completed or started by.

Tinea capitis – TIN-ee-uh kuh-PIY-tiss
– Commonly known as ringworm of the
scalp. The cause is a fungal, vegetable
parasite which infects the hair and skin.
It can be identified by circular grey or
white skin, surrounded by red, active
rings. The skin looks dull and rough. The
condition should be referred to a doctor.

Tinea corporis – TIN-ee-uh KOR-puh-riss – Ringworm of the body. A contagious fungal infection where there are circles of red itchy skin, which heal from the centre. On the scalp, it will result in hair loss.

Tinea cruris – TIN-ee-uh KROOuh-riss – A fungal infection that affects the groin area.

Tinea facei – TIN-ee-uh FAY-see-ay – A fungal infection that affects the face.

Tinea manuum – TIN-ee-uh MAN-yoo-uhm – A fungal infection that affects the hands.

Tinea pedis – TIN-ee-uh PED-iss – Commonly known as athlete's foot. The cause is a fungus that attacks the skin and can be identified by soft, sore skin, irritation, bleeding and a bad odour. The condition should be referred to a doctor.

Tinnitus – tin-IY-tuhss – Sensation of a ringing, roaring or buzzing sound in the ears or head, when no external sound is present.

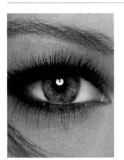

Tint colours – TINT KUH-luhz – Tubes of permanent dye that are designed to colour brow and lash hair. They are made for use around the delicate eye area and are activated by being mixed with hydrogen peroxide.

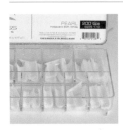

Tip – TIP – A plastic nail shape that is available in various shapes and sizes. It's applied to a natural nail and buffed to provide the length for the nail enhancement.

Tissue fluid – TISH-yoo FLOO-id – Often referred to as intercellular fluid, this is a watery substance that bathes all cells. It leaks into the blood capillaries and lymph capillaries.

Titanium dioxide – ti-TAY-nee-uhm diy-OK-siyd – A white mineral that provides a natural sun protection factor (SPF) to the skin.

Toner – TOH-nuh – A product that restores the skin's natural pH balance after it's been cleansed and removes any excess cleanser.

Tooth whitening – TOOTH WIYT-ning – A procedure to whiten and brighten the teeth.

Top coat – TOP koht – This coat of varnish gives a good shine to the nails and helps to make the coloured varnish last longer.

Topical hair growth – TOP-ikl HAIR GROHTH – Caused by an increase in blood supply to the area. It may result from plucking, waxing or wearing a plaster cast.

T

Topical (up-to-date) themes – TOP-ikl (UP-tuh-DAYT) THEEMZ – For example: football team colours, animals, superheroes, cultural occasions and combat camouflage.

Total intimate hair removal – TOH-tuhl IN -tim-uht HAIR ri-MOO-vuhl – All hair is removed from the lower back, buttocks, anus, scrotum and penis.

Total look – TOH-tuhl LUUK – The overall look. In the hair and beauty industry this includes hair, make-up and clothes.

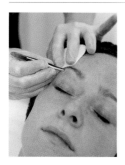

Total reshape – TOH-tuhl REE-shayp – A full treatment on the brows, changing the original shape completely.

Trades Description Act – TRAYDZ di-SKRIP-shuhn akt – The law stating that products should not falsely or misleadingly describe quality, fitness, price or purpose, by advertisements, displays or description.

Training and development plan – TRAY-ning uhnd duh-VEL-uhp-muhnt PLAN – A plan based on a therapist's weaknesses to help them build their confidence and skills.

Training providers – TRAY-ning pruh-VIY-duhz – Organisations that provide recognised training.

Transfers – TRANSS-furz – These are usually self-adhesive and can easily be applied to nails by first peeling off the backing sheet.

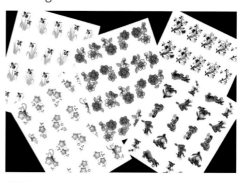

Transversally – tranz-VURSS-uh-lee – Across the nail, or along the width of the nail.

Transversus abdominus – tranz-VUR-suhss ab-DOM-i-nuhss – Muscle found deep on the anterior abdomen. It compresses the abdomen, keeping the abdominal organs in place.

Trapezius – truh-PEE-zee-uhss – Muscle that extends from the occipital bone across the shoulders towards the deltoids and midway down the back, attaching at the spine.

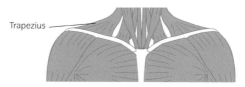

Trapezius

Treatment advice – TREET-muhnt uhd-VIYS – Recommendations given to the client following treatment to continue the benefits and prevent an unwanted contra-action.

Treatment objectives – TREET-muhnt uhb-JEK-tivz – The aims or desired end results of the treatment.

Treatment plan – TREET-muhnt PLAN – Stages you'll follow in carrying out a treatment. Include areas to be treated, type of treatment, contra-indications, contra-actions, advice, client signature and client feedback.

Triangularis – triy-ang-gyuh-LAH-riss/triy-ang-gyuh-LA-riss – Muscle that runs towards the neck from the corners of the mouth.

Triceps – TRIY-seps – Posterior upper arm muscle that extends and adducts the shoulder.

Trichotillomania – trik-uh-til-uh-MAY-nee-uh – A disorder or habit often triggered by stress or depression. Sufferers feel repeated urges to pull out scalp, lash, facial or brow hair, sometimes resulting in bald patches.

Trigger – TRIG-uh – Part of the airbrush used to regulate the spray.

Trigger point – TRIG-uh POYNT – A technique used in stone therapy to apply direct pressure to an isolated area. Often the side of the stone is used for this technique.

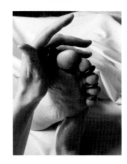

Tucking stones – TUK-ing STOHNZ – A technique used during a stone therapy treatment where the stones are tucked under the body or between the toes, fingers, etc.

Turbinate – TUR-bin-uht/TUR-bi-nayt – Two bones that form the outside of the nose.

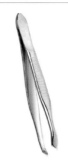

Tweezers – TWEE-zuhz – Made of stainless steel, these come in a variety of shapes: slanted, claw and pointed.

Two piece needle – TOO PEESS NEEDL – A needle made from two separate pieces of metal: the shank and the shaft. These have been crimped together and are used for hair removal methods of electrical epilation.

Typical salon reception duties – TIP-ikl SAL-o(ng) or suh-LO(ng) ri-SEP-shuhn DYOO-tiz – These include meeting and greeting clients, checking and making appointments, customer service, and promoting the sale of services and products.

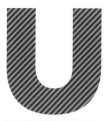

Ulna – UL-nuh – Bone located at the side of the forearm.

Ultraviolet light – UL-truh-VIY-uh-luht LIYT – Ultraviolet (UV) light consists of invisible rays of light, which are found in sunlight. Exposure to UV light can cause the skin to tan.

Ultraviolet radiation – UL-truh-VIY-uh-luht-ray-dee-AY-shuhn – A way of sterilising tools – remember to turn the tools over, so that each side is sterilised for at least 20 minutes.

Unique Selling Point (USP) – yoo-NEEK SEL-ing poynt -- YOO-ESS-PEE – Something which makes your product or service stand out from the competition's.

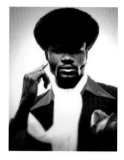

Unusual features – un-YOO-zhuhl FEE-chuhz – Extra care will be needed. These are features that need to be considered when determining the client's requirements. For example, when your client has dimples in the cheeks or chin when applying make-up. Other features to take care around are moles or the Adam's apple.

Up-selling – UP-SEL-ing – Recommending a product or service that isn't directly linked to a client's needs and expectations but will enhance their salon or home experience.

Upper arch – UP-uh AHCH – The curve of the nail from the base to the tip. A perfectly shaped nail has a gentle curve. Some people have flat nails, others have nails that can tilt upwards. These tend to be weaker than those with an upper arch curve.

Urethra – yoor-EETH-ruh – The narrow tube that runs through the length of the penis through which urine exits the body.

Urticaria

Urticaria – ur-ti-KAIR-ree-uh – Also known as hives or nettle rash, this is caused by exposure to an allergen, such as animal hair, food or latex. It's identified as an itchy rash with white bumps or weals that are surrounded by inflamed skin.

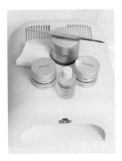

UV gel – YOO-VEE JEL – A thick gel that is cured into a hard, durable, flexible enhancement using a UV curing lamp.

UVA rays – YOO-VEE-AY RAYZ – These have a long wavelength and penetrate deep into the dermis, stimulating melanin production and causing a fast but short-lived tan. They are damaging to collagen and elastin, and lead to premature skin ageing.

UVB rays – YOO-VEE-BEE RAYZ – These penetrate to the lower levels of the epidermis to create a longer lasting tan. UVB stimulates Vitamin D production.

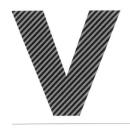

V

Vacuum suction – VAK-yoom SUK-shuhn – A treatment designed to stimulate lymphatic drainage, remove excess waste, reduce puffiness, and temporarily fill out fine lines and wrinkles.

Vapours – VAY-puhz – Chemical molecules in the air created by evaporation of a substance.

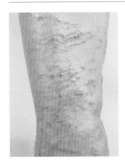

Varicose veins – VARR-i-kohss VAYNZ – Bulging surface veins that look blue/green and bulbous. They are caused by the valves in the veins breaking down, which results in a stagnation of blood and causes obstruction, making the veins bulge.

Vasoconstriction of blood vessels – VASS-oh-kuhn-STRIK-shuhn or VAY-zoh-kuhn-STRIK-shuhn uhv BLUD VESS-uhlz – The narrowing of the blood vessels, allowing less blood to flow. This usually occurs when the body gets cold and the vital organs need the blood more than the skin.

Vasodilation of blood vessels – VASS-oh-diy-LAY-shuhn or VAY-zoh-diy-LAY-shuhn uhv BLUD VESS-uhlz – The widening of the blood vessels, allowing more blood to flow. This usually occurs when the body gets hot and can be seen by the red colour of the skin.

Vastus intermedius, lateralis and medialis – VASS-tuhss in-tuh-MEE-dee-uhss, la-tuh-RAY-liss uhnd mee-dee-AY-liss – Three muscles that form part of the group called the quadriceps. They run down the front of the leg from the femur to the tibia and extend the knee.

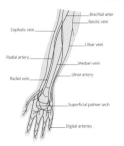

Vein – VAYN – Transports mainly deoxygenated blood from the cells and tissues.

Vellus hair – VEL-uhss HAIR – Soft, fine downy hair found on the face and body.

Ventilation – ven-ti-LAY-shuhn – Keeping the treatment room free of vapours or harmful sprays.

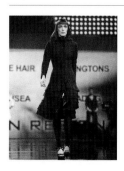

Venue – VEN-yoo – The place where a promotional event is held; it might be at the local theatre, for instance.

Venule – VEN-yoo-uhl or VEEN-yoo-uhl – A small blood vessel that allows deoxygenated blood to return from the capillaries to the veins.

Verbal – VUR-buhl – Use of the voice to communicate with the client.

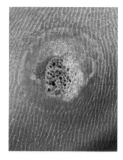

Verruca – vuh-ROO-kuh – A wart on the sole or toes of the foot. The virus attacks the skin through direct contact, generally from walking on moist surfaces, eg showers or swimming pool floors.

Vibrations – viy-BRAY-shuhnz – Trembling movements that can stimulate or relax the nerves depending on how they are applied.

Viral infection – VIY-ruhl in-FEK-shuhn – Any type of infection caused by a virus.

Virus – VIY-ruhss – Viruses are too small to be seen with the eye; they can only be seen under a microscope. They are easily spread by coughing, sneezing and touching.

Viscosity – viss-KOSS-it-ee – The density of a liquid.

Vitamins – VIT-uh-minz – Fat or water-soluble organic substances, essential for normal growth and activity of the body. They are obtained naturally from plant and animal foods.

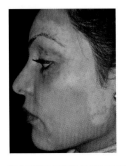

Vitiligo – vi-ti-LIY-goh or vi-ti-LEE-goh – A hypo-pigmentation disorder resulting in areas of very pale skin, with little or no pigment present.

Vocational qualifications – vuh-KAY-shuhn-uhl kwol-if-i-KAY-shuhnz – A vocational qualification gives people the skills an employer is looking for. These work-related qualifications let you learn in the way that suits you.

Volatility – vo-luh-TIL-it-ee – The speed at which an essential oil evaporates.

Voluntary muscles – VOL-uhn-tree MUSSLZ – Muscles that are controlled by the brain.

Vomer – VOH-muh – Bone that forms the nasal septum.

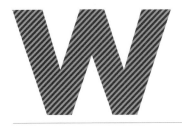

Warm wax – WORM WAKS N.B. 'warm' rhymes with 'form' – A type of warm cream or liquid wax which is applied thinly with a spatula in the direction of the hair growth. Paper or muslin cloth is then pressed on and the strip is removed against the hair growth.

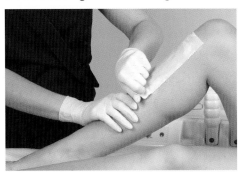

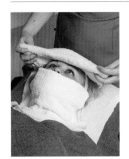

Warming devices – WORM-ing di-VIY-siz N.B. 'warming' rhymes with 'forming' – These include steam, hot towels or hot damp pads that are used to open the hair follicles to make the removal of the hairs easier.

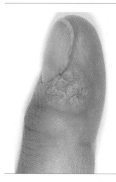

Warts – WORTS N.B. 'warts' rhymes with 'forts' – A viral infection commonly found on the hands. They look raised with a rough surface and a flat top.

Waste materials – WAYST muh-TEER-ree-uhlz – Used items that need to be thrown away after the service is completed.

Waste products – WAYST PROD-uhkts – Packaging that may be left over at the end of the service and must be disposed of correctly.

Water erosion – WOR-tuh i-ROH-zhuhn – Gradual wearing away of material caused by the action of water.

Water hardness – WOR-tuh HARD-niss – The level of calcium present in the water, which, if high, can cause corrosion, staining and scaling.

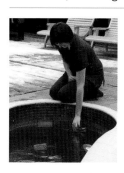

Water testing kit – WOR-tuh TESS-ting kit – Method for testing and maintaining the quality of water in the spa area.

Water-based make-up – WOR-tuh-BAYSST MAYK-up – Dries to a natural matte finish that is neither drier nor shinier in appearance than skin is naturally.

Wax application and removal techniques – WAKS ap-li-KAY-shuhn uhnd ri-MOO-vuhl tek-NEEKS – These will differ according to the waxing system used. Always follow manufacturer's instructions.

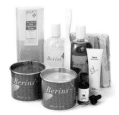

Wax depilation – WAKS de-pi-LAY-shuhn – The removal of unwanted hair from a body part (using wax), which will grow back in approximately four weeks.

Wax strips – WAKS STRIPS – Made of either paper or fabric and placed on the warm wax to remove it from the skin.

Waxing – WAK-sing – The use of wax to remove unwanted hairs temporarily, from the face or body.

Ways of communicating – WAYZ uhv kum-MYOO-ni-KAY-ting – These include verbal (how you speak) and non-verbal (body language, writing, listening).

When to refer problems – WEN tuh ri-FUR PROB-luhmz – You will need to refer problems to a senior member of staff when the problems are outside your own level of responsibility.

Whiplash – WIP-lash – A condition produced when the muscles, ligaments, discs or nerves in the neck region are damaged due to sudden trauma. Indian head massage can help to relieve pain and discomfort.

Working co-operatively – WUR-king koh-OP-uh-ri-tiv-lee – Being helpful and supportive of your team.

Working patterns – WUR-king PAT-uhnz – The hours that an employee will work, for example part-time, full-time, or shift work.

Working safely – WUR-king SAYF-lee – You must make sure you follow the COSHH regulations (store, handle, use and dispose) when working with chemicals. Always comply with the health and safety regulations and follow instructions carefully.

Working Time Directive – WUR-king TIYM duh-REK-tiv – Your right not to have to work more than 48 hours a week on average, unless you choose to or work in a sector with its own rules. Your normal working hours should be set out in your employment contract or written statement of employment particulars.

Workplace policy – WUK-playss POL-iss-ee – Your salon will have rules about various procedures relating to health and safety, eg COSHH Regulations referring to the use of chemicals. These policies are often recorded in an employee handbook.

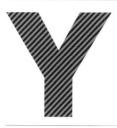

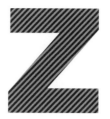

Y Lashes – WY LASH-iz – Lashes that split in two at the tapered end. This gives the effect of double the amount of lashes. They can be applied in half the normal time.

Zinc oxide – ZINK OK-siyd – A white mineral with a more opaque tone that provides light-reflecting qualities.

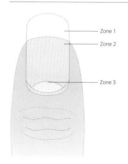

Zone 1
Zone 2
Zone 3

Zones – ZOHNZ – Areas of the nail plate that are split into three sections: Zone one – the free edge; Zone two – the apex area; Zone three – the cuticle area.

Zygomatic – zi-guh-MAT-ik/ziy-guh-MAT-ik – Two bones that form the cheekbones.

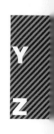

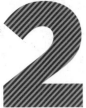

2

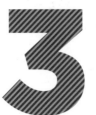

3

2D surface – too-DEE SUR-fiss – A design that has been applied to paper.

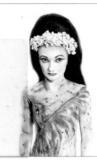

3D surface – three-DEE SUR-fiss – A design that has been applied to the body, mannequin or nail plate.

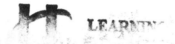